A practical, drug-free alternative guide to combating Psoriasis. This book is intended to help anyone with Psoriasis no matter how chronic or advanced and is packed full of innovative and diverse information.

The remedies and methods contained within this book are a combination of things that have been observed to help even the most stubborn Psoriasis cases. Where possible, scientific evidence is given for the reasoning behind what is suggested.

For more information please visit:
www.parhamdonyai.com
www.reflexology.co.uk

Published by:
Active Press
*a subsidiary of Active Worldwide Limited*

Please contact:
info@active.gi

*To those who seek answers and are determined enough to overcome life's obstacles.*

# Prologue

There is a "cure" for every disease right here on earth. The problem is, we are not inquisitive enough, we are not lucky enough, we don't look in the right places, we don't ask the right questions, we don't come across the right people, we are not open minded enough or sometimes we just run out of patience or time.

Psoriasis is incurable according to doctors. Many diseases are incurable according to doctors. After all, if many diseases would be cured with a simple vitamin or lifestyle change, where would the pharmaceutical industry make its billions from?

For some, illness is profit. Curing it means no profit.

I am not saying there is a conspiracy; just convenience. This book is about remedies and methods that will help heal your Psoriasis right now - today. If you want to see a significant reduction in your Psoriasis, put the first 3 recommendations into action for a noticeable improvement. If your Psoriasis gets a great deal better but is not 100% gone, then start implementing the other recommendations that follow.

Don't be concerned with the past and why no one has told you these. It doesn't matter. You are here now. Let's make today the first day of your journey to be rid of Psoriasis or at least see a substantial reduction in its appearance and the effects it has on your life.

Please note that I am not a doctor and don't profess to be. All the advice given in this book is NOT intended to replace sound medical advice and is not a replacement for traditional medicine. If you are on any medication, do not stop it and seek the advice of your doctor before you make any changes. This applies in particular to oral steroid medication which many Psoriasis sufferers are on.

There IS a way to substantially reduce your Psoriasis. There is also a way for you to totally eliminate it. How much you progress is very much dependant on your determination and the severity of your Psoriasis.

Many of the answers to alleviating Psoriasis lie within the following pages. If you do not see the results expected, come back to the first chapter and start reading the book again. You may have missed something.

Healing Psoriasis and the advice in this book is an ongoing journey for me as a researcher and author and I always look to update things when a new discovery is made or when I am made aware of something useful. If you wish to update me of your progress, your feedback, your before/after photos, please do so. That way, future issues of this book can contain updates. You can send these to the email of my publishers: info@active.gi.

The best of luck to you and the best of health to you.

Parham Donyai
2023

# The TOP 3 things which will immediately help improve your skin health and reduce the symptoms of Psoriasis

I am not going to waste your time by telling you what Psoriasis is. There are other books for that and if you or a loved one have Psoriasis, then you already know what it is.

As I write this book, the reality is that the medical profession does not know what Psoriasis really is or how to "cure" it. I use the word cure with some trepidation, because not many diseases are in actual fact cured, unless they are of a bacterial nature and you take antibiotics.

What the medical profession does know about Psoriasis is that it is an auto-immune disorder.

But what exactly causes this auto-immune disorder?

In my job as a complimentary medicine practitioner, I am more concerned with causes than anything else, because if you can find the cause, then in theory you can in most cases find the cure. I say causes (plural) on purpose as quite often with diseases which have a complex nature, the cause is often more than one.

I also use the terms "in my job" loosely because whilst I have been qualified in complimentary medicine for some 30 years, it has not been a full time occupation.

If I was to break down what has taken most of my time over the last 30 years, it has been the formulation and manufacturing of nutritional supplements, setting up various businesses, writing and mentoring individuals.

Whilst unrelated to Psoriasis, being in the fitness, health and nutrition "industry" as it were, alongside dealing with people in need of help with their ailments, has given me an interesting angle. Combine this with my aerial view of things, I am sure you will find some, if not all the things in the following pages very useful and extremely helpful as far as Psoriasis is concerned.

What you will find in the following pages are quite a few scientific references to the relevant points I raise to give you the reasoning behind them. Feel free to read them or not. I usually put them at the end of each paragraph for ease of finding them.

You will be most surprised to read that the main parts of this book are served very early on, in that I will tell you THE top 3 most effective ways to immediately bring your

Psoriasis under significant control and see a clear reduction usually within a few weeks and without changing much in your life.

Some people see a total alleviation of their Psoriasis in days - depending on many factors including the severity of their Psoriasis and the duration they have been suffering with it. I am not promising this to YOU. Just saying that some people DO see this sort of crazy healing from a disease they have been burdened with for years.

Most people want to cure ailments but they are not prepared to pay the price. They are not willing to change their lifestyle, habits or diets.

You don't have to make all the changes in this book, which may put you off the journey and ensure you do not stick to the regime!

If you are like most people, whenever you do something that is too dramatic and requires too much effort, you will probably not stick to it.

Us humans are so simple and predictable! That is why most of us are burdened with our long term problems and very few ultra-determined individuals truly conquer disease.

If you truly want to conquer your Psoriasis to a great extent and possibly totally eradicate it, I will tell you how to do that, and guess what? I know, you are going to be surprised but I will tell you right now. Yes, in the next paragraph:

*If you truly want to conquer your Psoriasis, you need to dramatically change your diet to a plant-based diet where 80% of your diet is vegetables/ salads and 20% is vegetable proteins and good fats, add an 18+6 intermittent fasting regime, avoid the nightshade vegetables, avoid refined sugar, avoid peanuts and drink lots of water.*

See, I told you that you won't stick to it! Not most of you anyway. Most people find the above too much of a big change and even if they start doing it, they don't stick to it.

"Curing" Psoriasis for most people is as simple as the above. Change your diet to a vegetarian one, avoid sugar, avoid meat, all junk, fried foods, avoid certain vegetables that are in the nightshade family, avoid dairy, avoid wheat, avoid peanuts, avoid oats and drink lots of water. Throw in some intermittent fasting and hey presto, your skin will be back to being how it was supposed to be.

Now, you are going to tell me what a waste of money this book was because the advice came in the first few lines and the rest was just fillers. Maybe. Depends on you. If you are serious and bothered enough, then yes this aforementioned advice is pretty much all you need.

However, having worked with people as a mentor, as a complimentary medicine practitioner, as a businessman and so on, I know for a fact that few people will actually change their diets that dramatically. As bothersome as

Psoriasis is, most people learn to live with it and most people are too busy, too tired, too lazy, too stressed etc etc to actually try this change in diet or more likely, to stick to it... for life! Yes I did say for life and that is probably where even fewer people stick to the regime.

If you get your Psoriasis under control, you can have some of the things you love periodically but in moderation.

You can of course try various dietary changes for a while and see good results but with a genetic problem like Psoriasis, chances are that it will come back as soon as you go back to your old ways.

Genetics have loaded the gun with the Psoriasis gene in your case and your lifestyle and habits are what pushes the trigger.

Elon Musk recently put it in an interesting way. He said he rather enjoy his life, do what he wants and die young than stick to all these different workouts and regimes for staying healthy!

That can work too but I am guessing if you are reading this book, you don't share his philosophy!

This book is a balance. It is about not going too crazy with changing your entire diet (unless you want to or there is a severe need to - such as very stubborn Psoriasis) but at the same time about giving you solid advice about certain things that are causing and/or making your Psoriasis worse and how you can see a huge improvement by making small changes.

I am going to devote a short section to each thing that can make a big difference to your Psoriasis. I will list them in order of importance.

In other words, the most important ones that will make the most difference to your Psoriasis are going to be the first things I will mention. They will be the first 3 things in fact.

What I ask in return for the advice coming up is that you DO stick to at least the first 2 things coming up and you give them a fair shot, such as 2 months. If in addition to the first 2 main things, if you want to go on a vegetarian diet of salads and vegetables for a while, you will only see better and quicker results - but this is not absolutely necessary to see significant improvements.

The first 2 major points will have a significant positive impact on your Psoriasis but may not totally eradicate it. If so and yours is a stubborn case, then you need to make the additional dietary changes. However for most people, the first 2 points are enough to make them happy and change their life for the better.

If you have Psoriasis, I know you may have been conned before. This is the problem with chronic disease. You will come across a lot of cons before you come across something that actually works. There are a lot of people out there wanting to make money out of desperate and emotional people.

At this stage you may be wondering if I know the cause of Psoriasis. The actual cause. The answer is yes and no. We know that it is an auto-immune disorder but what triggers it? At the end of the day, many people have many bad disease genes that never get triggered. Many siblings have the same cancer genes, but only some of them get cancer. What triggers Psoriasis in people and how come some people have it all their lives, others get it periodically and for some other lucky ones, it goes away as spontaneously as it appeared? Some very lucky ones have the gene but never get Psoriasis!

If you take the simple fact that a rather dramatic change in diet can make your Psoriasis virtually disappear and as long as you stick to this diet, it won't come back, then you have your answer, don't you?

Psoriasis comes from the intestinal and digestive system. In fact, many complimentary medicine practitioners believe that Psoriasis is the body's way of throwing out substances it cannot deal with in the digestive system into the bloodstream. It literally throws them out - onto the skin.

But you know Psoriasis is not as simple as that and the gut connection does not explain fully certain things like how sunshine reduces the severity of Psoriasis and how a simple £500 home device can in some cases eliminate it in some people (more on this coming up).

Psoriasis is complex but not totally elusive and there are ways to manage it or at least reduce its potency by so much that it will no longer be a huge concern in your life. For many, you can in fact cure yourself of it.

The methods in this book are the "alternative" methods to the traditional medical ones.

A doctor will willingly tell you that s/he cannot cure your Psoriasis. They can only diagnose, suppress and control it to a certain extent. Traditional cures for Psoriasis can come with side effects and you may find that you are having to go to more and more extreme measures to suppress it.

In some stubborn cases, you may even want to combine traditional ways of combating Psoriasis with what I am going to share with you in this book; at least at the outset until you see significant improvements. I am not anti-doctor. It is just that if they can't cure something, surely logic would dictate for you to find alternatives that can or at least may heal your skin.

The traditional methods of combating Psoriasis are not cures but they can help. This is why I am mentioning them in this book but they will be all the way at the end!

Do remember that "suppressing" Psoriasis is not a cure and more often than not it can cause more long term harm and dependency. However I totally get that some people need drugs or other alternatives and you need to do what is best for you.

# Number 0: Before we get going

This one is not in the top 3 because for most people, it is not easy to do.

All the things coming up in this book are on the assumption that you cannot and/or will not move country! Because one of the most effective ways to substantially reduce your Psoriasis and possibly totally eliminate it is to move to a sunny country AND be near the sea, bathe in the sea regularly and then catch a few hours of sun afterwards.

After a few weeks of doing this, your Psoriasis will disappear but you will need to keep going into the sea and catching sun to keep it at bay.

This simple, yet unreachable for most people, lifestyle change can alleviate the majority of Psoriasis cases.

**The Dead Sea**

Many people go to the Dead Sea in Jordan or Israel to cure their Psoriasis, as it is believed the high concentration of salt in that region combined with a special sun is a cure-all for Psoriasis. These same people would get very similar benefits if they devoted as much time as they do in the Dead Sea to bathing in any sea and catching some sun. The salts of the Dead Sea possibly act as catalysts or maybe they get rid of the hard Psoriasis skin faster. There is no doubt that the Dead Sea is a strange and peculiar place.

I have been to the Dead Sea and there is so much salt in there that you basically float! Heaven help you if you have a cut because that salt stings!

The Dead Sea is unlike any other body of water on Earth. It contains a high concentration of minerals, including magnesium, calcium, potassium, and bromide, which are essential for the skin's health. Notably, the magnesium levels in the Dead Sea are about fifteen times higher than salts in other seas.

Research suggests that the minerals found in the Dead Sea have significant anti-inflammatory effects. We will mention "inflammation" a lot in this book because Psoriasis in many ways is inflammation. If you can reduce the inflammation internally or externally, you are on a good path.

A study published in the Journal of Investigative Dermatology found that bathing in the magnesium-rich Dead Sea salt solution significantly improved skin barrier function and reduced inflammation in patients with atopic dry skin (Proksch et al., 2005). We will talk about skin barrier a fair bit in this book.

The Dead Sea is located more than 400 meters below sea level, the lowest point on the earth's surface. The unique location results in a filtering of the sun's UV rays. This means that the UVB light reaching the area is less harmful but still effective for treating skin conditions like Psoriasis. Research published in Clinical Dermatology found that UVB Phototherapy is a highly effective treatment for Psoriasis (Palmieri et al., 2007).

The Dead Sea reduces inflammation. Reducing inflammation will aid or eliminate Psoriasis but it is not a cure. The problem is still there if one accepts that it is a gut problem (more later), but if something reduces all the inflammation, then you could consider it a cure. However, although going to the Dead Sea may temporarily fix your Psoriasis, it will not cure it for life.

You are likely to see your Psoriasis back when you move away from the Dead Sea or any sea, usually within weeks.

Dead Sea Climatotherapy involves a combination of sun exposure (Phototherapy) and bathing in the sea. A study published in the Journal of the American Academy of Dermatology showed significant improvements in Psoriasis patients following a course of Dead Sea Climatotherapy, with the benefits lasting for several months (Abels et al., 2008). Note: several months, not years or a lifetime.

The remaining people who may not benefit from sea and sun as much, are the hardcore Psoriasis sufferers that do a LOT of things wrong and there are many of them by the way! It may even be you, but don't worry, we will address some other things you can do to help yourself later on in the book.

With the above out of the way, let's get going with what will give you a noticeable improvement in your Psoriasis.

# Number 1: Vitamin D Oral Supplementation

Throughout history, many diseases confounded physicians and brought devastation to populations. It wasn't until the discovery of specific vitamins and minerals that the root causes of these illnesses were unveiled and treated. The impact of these micronutrients on health is profound, and their introduction into diets has virtually eradicated several once-common diseases. Let's dive into some of these conditions and the vitamins and minerals that proved pivotal in their treatment.

## 1. Scurvy and Vitamin C

Scurvy, characterised by bleeding gums, joint pain, and anaemia, was particularly common among sailors during long voyages.

British naval surgeon James Lind discovered in the 18th century that citrus fruits like lemons and oranges could prevent and cure scurvy. It was later identified that the vital component was Vitamin C (Ascorbic Acid). A simple glass of orange juice would have helped eliminate Scurvy!

The British Navy adopted lemon or lime juice as a mandatory inclusion in sailors' diets, effectively eliminating scurvy from its ranks.
Reference: Carpenter, K. J. 1986. "The history of scurvy and vitamin C." Cambridge University Press.


## 2. Rickets and Vitamin D

Rickets leads to soft, weak bones in children, resulting in deformities and bone pain. It was once rampant in urban areas of Europe and North America.

In the early 20th century, it was found that cod liver oil and exposure to ultraviolet light could prevent and cure rickets. These were sources of Vitamin D, which is crucial for calcium absorption and bone health.

Many countries began fortifying milk and other foods with Vitamin D, leading to a significant decline in rickets cases.

Reference: Pettifor, J. M. 2014. "Nutritional rickets: pathogenesis and prevention." Pediatric Endocrinology Reviews.


## 3. Pellagra and Niacin (Vitamin B3)

Pellagra is marked by the four D's: dermatitis, diarrhea, dementia, and death! Yikes! It was once widespread in the American South.

In the early 20th century, Dr. Joseph Goldberger demonstrated that pellagra was linked to diet. Later, it was found that niacin (Vitamin B3) deficiency was the culprit.

With the introduction of niacin-rich foods and niacin fortification, pellagra cases dramatically decreased.
Reference: Bollet, A. J. 1992. "Politics and pellagra: the epidemic of Pellagra in the U.S. in the early twentieth century." The Yale Journal of Biology and Medicine.


## 4. Goiter and Iodine

Goiter is an enlargement of the thyroid gland, leading to a prominent swelling in the neck. It was prevalent in regions with iodine-deficient soils.

In the early 20th century, it was established that iodine was essential for thyroid function and that its deficiency led to Goiter.

Many countries initiated iodine fortification of salt, which substantially reduced the incidence of Goiter.

Reference: Zimmermann, M. B., & Boelaert, K. 2015. "Iodine deficiency and thyroid disorders." The Lancet Diabetes & Endocrinology.

There are many other examples that may not be generally known or written in history books, such as Magnesium for morning sickness.

The relationship between certain diseases and micronutrient deficiencies serves as a testament to the importance of balanced nutrition or the need for extra nutrition in some cases. The introduction of a single vitamin or mineral has, in several instances, been the turning point in combating debilitating diseases. These historical lessons emphasise the significance of ongoing research in nutrition and its potential to transform public health.

However, sometimes this research is not beneficial to the big Pharmaceutical Companies making money out of disease.

So we come to the saviour of Rickets, but in much bigger doses. This knight in shining armour is Vitamin D.

There is no doubt that Vitamin D supplementation greatly helps Psoriasis. <u>We are talking Vitamin D3 here</u>.

Vitamin D comes from the sun and anyone with Psoriasis will know that when they go in the sun, their Psoriasis improves.

The problem is that often they are not in the sun long enough or that the sun doesn't reach their actual problematic skin because of dry skin on top of healthy skin or both!

Most people go on holiday for a couple of weeks a year and that is just not enough if you have Psoriasis. Even if you live in a sunny country, you may not go out and about regularly with your whole body exposed.

The second issue is that for the sun to work, you need the problematic area to be free of that extra thick dry layer of skin caused by Psoriasis. You need the sun to fully penetrate the top layer of your skin for it to start healing your Psoriasis.

Please note that if you have very red and inflamed skin, you will want to start exposing it to the sun very slowly and in small amounts. You can also try putting sunscreen to reduce the severity of the sun on exposed skin, until it starts slowly healing and getting better. You don't want to go from Psoriasis to skin cancer! So, it is much better to be cautious and start slowly but surely. Putting anything on the skin such as sunscreen is not ideal (more later) but again, we need to reach a balance.

Even if you have managed to get rid of that top dry layer (more later) and you get some sun, if you are eating and drinking a whole load of offending foods (also more later), your relief will be short lived.

Vitamin D modulates the body's immune response, which is a key element in the pathogenesis of Psoriasis.

According to the Journal of Clinical & Cellular Immunology, Vitamin D can inhibit the proliferation of pro-inflammatory cells that play a role in the development of Psoriasis (Mora, Iwata, & von Andrian, 2008).

Psoriasis is characterised by an abnormal growth of Keratinocytes, the predominant cell type in the outer layer of skin. According to a study published in The Journal of Investigative Dermatology, Vitamin D analogs can regulate the growth and differentiation of Keratinocytes (Bikle, 2011).

***Simply put, Vitamin D supplementation can regulate your Psoriasis!***

Oral vitamin D supplementation has scientifically been shown to have benefits in Psoriasis. A study published in Dermato-Endocrinology found that oral Vitamin D supplementation improved Psoriasis symptoms in patients with low baseline Vitamin D levels (Finamor et al., 2013). Dosages in these studies vary, but a common starting dose is 1000 to 2000 IU daily, often adjusted based on blood levels of 25-Hydroxyvitamin D, the indicator of Vitamin D status.

By the way, you may be sitting there thinking "oh, well, I don't have low baseline Vitamin D"! I can almost guarantee you that you do! A simple blood test can give you the result.

You probably already know that topical Vitamin D can help your Psoriasis. Topical vitamin D analogs, such as Calcipotriol and Calcitriol, are commonly used to treat mild to moderate Psoriasis. According to a review published in

the American Journal of Clinical Dermatology, these agents
have been found to be effective and safe for treating
Psoriasis (van de Kerkhof, et al., 2011). The typical dosage
for Calcipotriol is usually up to 100g per week, and for
Calcitriol is usually 30g to 100g per week.


For our purposes, we are NOT talking about topical
Vitamin D that comes in the form of creams, gels and
lotions. We are talking about oral Vitamin D that you can
ingest.

In fact, topical Vitamin D has a nasty side effect for many
in that it can turn your skin permanently darker. So, you
use it, get rid of your Psoriasis temporarily (it is not a cure)
but end up with a permanent dark area on your body -
possibly as unsightly as Psoriasis patches for some! This is a
serious side effect and even more long-lasting than Psoriasis
that most doctors don't tell you! Be careful using Vitamin D
creams!


Vitamin D from the sun can possibly cure your Psoriasis
if not for several factors such as not getting enough sun, not
getting it regularly and/or the rest of your lifestyle
countering any positive effects. i.e eating bad and reducing
the effects of the sun exposure.


As the first part of your Psoriasis healing plan, please go
to the health shop or go online and purchase a good brand
Vitamin D supplement. Don't go for the cheapest. Go for

something with good reviews. It needs to be a high dose one.

You need to start taking anywhere between 4000IU and 20,000 IU daily.

Vitamin D is a fat soluble vitamin, so generally you don't want to be taking too much of it.

Most people, even in sunny countries are Vitamin D deficient; it seems that people with Psoriasis are particularly Vitamin D deficient.

The Recommended Daily Amount (RDA) of Vitamin D for an adult is 600IU which is 15 Micrograms. This is just not enough if you have Psoriasis.

The problem with taking excess Vitamin D is that it may give you side effects and doctors don't generally recommend it.  However, it has been argued that people can take as much as 20,000 IU a day for years without side effects. Everyone is different.

If you have Psoriasis, I would suggest you start taking 4000 IU a day immediately. See how you get on with it for around 7 days and pay very close attention to your various Psoriatic areas.

If there is a huge improvement, stick to 4000 IU a day. If there is no difference at all, up it to 10,000 IU a day. If you start seeing a marked difference in your skin after 7 days, stick to 10,000 IU a day.

If yours is a stubborn case, you can go up to 20,000 IU a day. Do not go over this amount. At 20,000 IU a day, you are extremely likely to notice an improvement in your Psoriasis.

This book is not a one directional piece of work. I am very much interested in your feedback and what has worked for you.

What you are being told is what has been working for many people up to now.

Excess Vitamin D may give you side effects, so you need to monitor and see how you feel. For example 10,000 IU and above per day may give the feeling of a tight chest when you breathe in. This is the case for a tiny minority of people but when I have spoken to them, they are not that bothered as they see their skin healing!

I will always advise you to do high dose Vitamin D supplementation at these levels with the assistance or approval of your doctor. I am also too aware that many doctors will dismiss it and tell you that these levels of Vitamin D will harm you or not do anything for your Psoriasis.

Remember, doctors are not trained in nutrition!

The role of nutrition in promoting health and preventing disease is undeniable. Chronic diseases such as diabetes, cardiovascular diseases, obesity, and even some cancers have clear links to dietary habits. Yet, surprisingly, the importance of nutrition is often underemphasised in modern medical education. This discrepancy raises the question: Are doctors adequately prepared to address the nutritional roots of today's health challenges? And this is why I say, please take the advice of your doctor but remember, they are not trained to advise you on nutrition for health!

Medical students in many countries receive less than 25 hours of nutrition instruction over their entire medical school career, a fraction of the overall curriculum!

Nutrition often gets bundled with other subjects, reducing the focus it receives.
Reference: Adams, K. M., Kohlmeier, M., & Zeisel, S. H. 2010. "Nutrition education in U.S. medical schools: latest update of a national survey." Academic Medicine.

While student doctors may learn the basics of biochemistry and physiology related to nutrition, translating that knowledge into practical dietary advice for patients can be challenging due to limited training.

Diets high in processed foods, sugars, and unhealthy fats are associated with a range of chronic diseases.

On the contrary, diets rich in whole foods, fruits, vegetables, and lean proteins can prevent or even reverse certain conditions.
Reference: Hu, F. B. 2002. "Dietary pattern analysis: a new direction in nutritional epidemiology."

For conditions like type 2 diabetes, nutritional interventions can be as effective as medications. Similarly, heart disease, the leading cause of death globally, has strong ties to dietary habits.

Recognising and addressing nutritional deficiencies or poor dietary habits early can prevent the onset of many chronic conditions.
Reference: Estruch, R., Ros, E., Salas-Salvadó, J., et al. 2013. "Primary Prevention of Cardiovascular Disease with a Mediterranean Diet Supplemented with Extra-Virgin Olive Oil or Nuts." New England Journal of Medicine.

Without a solid grounding in nutrition, doctors might miss the chance to guide their patients toward healthier dietary choices, relying instead solely on medication. They can also just not be informed when you take something that's new to them, such as high doses of Vitamin D. They do not have the experience, training or patient records to guide you.

While dieticians specialise in nutrition, they're not always integrated into general healthcare settings, limiting patients' access to expert dietary advice.

Patients often expect dietary guidance from their doctors. When physicians aren't equipped to provide this, there may be missed opportunities for preventive care.

It is your body and your choice at the end of the day. Psoriasis is your body telling you that there is something wrong already! If Vitamin D supplementation heals your Psoriasis, then you can come to your own conclusions.

Excess Vitamin D's main side effect is the build-up of calcium in your body which can cause nausea, vomiting, weakness, frequent urination. If you notice any of these, then you want to either reduce the dosage or stop. This is really up to you and your doctor.

Please don't put this book down all petrified and not wanting to carry on! The possibility of side effects with even 20,000 IU of Vitamin D a day for years is very slim. What you are more than likely going to experience is a gradual eradication of your Psoriasis, which is why you are reading this book and why I have put this route as the number 1 aid to healing your Psoriasis. Most importantly it is a route with minimum disruption to your lifestyle.

Once you see results or total elimination, you can stop or reduce the dosage, knowing that you can try this route again any time your Psoriasis gets out of control again.

Some of you may have tried Vitamin D before and not had great success. This will most likely be due to 3 reasons:

One, you did not take a high enough dosage. Most vitamin companies sell the bare minimum, something like 100 IU. This is nothing! It is nowhere near enough to see results even if you take 10 of their pills daily.

Two, you didn't take enough and/or enough for long enough. You need to give Vitamin D a chance to start working and this may be up to a month for some people. You must not skip a dose.

Three, you didn't buy a reputable brand. Much like everything else in life, you get good and bad. Just because a company says they have Vitamin D, it does not mean they have spent the money or have the capabilities to give you the good stuff! I am sorry to disappoint you if you thought all companies are equal!

It is suggested for you to read reviews on various Vitamin D3 supplements and choose one with good reviews and obviously one that comes in a high enough dosage for you to be able to take at least 4000 IU and possibly 4-5 times that a day.

***If you take a good brand of Vitamin D3, around 10,000 IU every day, you will see an improvement in your Psoriasis.***

There is a fair number of scientific data on Vitamin D and Psoriasis but please do remember that it is NOT in the interests of the Pharmaceutical Industry for you to be able to cure or substantially reduce your Psoriasis with a £10 bottle of vitamin!!!

Some studies below, if you are interested:

Mora, J. R., Iwata, M., & von Andrian, U. H. (2008). Vitamin effects on the immune system: vitamins A and D take centre stage. Journal of Clinical & Cellular Immunology, 134(2), 978-985.

Bikle, D. (2011). Vitamin D: Production, Metabolism, and Mechanisms of Action. In Endotext [Internet].

MDText.com, Inc.

Finamor, D. C., et al. (2013). A pilot study assessing the effect of prolonged administration of high daily doses of vitamin D on the clinical course of vitiligo and Psoriasis. Dermato-Endocrinology, 5(1), 222-234.

# Number 2: Soft water

I don't know where you live but it potentially has a direct link to you having Psoriasis and to the severity of your Psoriasis.

You may say that Psoriasis is caused by a gene. Yes, you need to have the gene but a lot more needs to happen before it gets triggered and stays triggered!

If you live in a hard water area, your Psoriasis will be much worse. If you live in a soft water area, your Psoriasis will be milder.

Read this again:

***If you live in a hard water area, your Psoriasis will be much worse. If you live in a soft water area, your Psoriasis will be milder!***

In fact, have you ever noticed your skin getting better or worse when you go on holiday somewhere or if you stay in another location for a while? You may have put it down to stress or lack of stress?

Unless for some reason you don't bathe or come into contact with water, you will be under its influence especially when it comes to Psoriasis.

Hard water makes Psoriasis much worse. The harder the water, the worse the Psoriasis and vice versa.

I will give you a personal example:

I never had Psoriasis, though I had the gene from my dad's side. A combination of eating a lot of sweets (we bought a sweet shop for a short while) and taking several courses of antibiotics in my early twenties triggered the gene. I started getting mild and sometimes moderate Psoriasis. I was living in London at the time.

A bit further on in life, I bought a flat in Marbella, Spain which had a massive industrial water softener for the whole block.

Whenever I would stay in the flat in Marbella, I would see the Psoriasis patches disappearing, especially when it was hotter and I could bathe in the sea also.

In fact, the water softener was so noticeable as a healer for Psoriasis that on one visit to Marbella, I noticed my skin was not getting any better - as had been the case on each prior visit.

I spoke to the gardener of the block and asked him if the water softener was working because I didn't think it was. He was astonished! He said it had stopped working and they were trying to fix it. He couldn't figure out how I knew!

This is how noticeable the effects of the water softener were!

Returning to London meant problem skin if I didn't keep my diet in check, so I installed a water softener in my house in London. It wasn't as powerful as the Marbella one, but it did the job.

Marbella was hassle-free as I didn't have to change salt or do anything. When you have one installed in your house, you do need to be on top of the salt and yes, it does cost.

I own several properties. One of them is in Lisbon, where the water is very hard in places.

When I would go to Lisbon, my property was in the outskirts and it had probably the hardest water I have ever seen. Within 1-2 days of being in Lisbon, no matter what else I brought under control, my skin would become inflamed and look terrible. My fingers looked like the skin was falling off of them.

So, Marbella with its softened water would heal Psoriasis and Lisbon with its extreme hard water would exacerbate Psoriasis - all other things remaining the same.

Nothing else that I did countered this rapid inflammation and worsening of my skin in Lisbon apart from number 1 above, high dose Vitamin D supplementation. However no natter how much Vitamin D supplementation I took, the hard water was just too much of a problem.

I would be better than if not taking the Vitamin D but I wasn't fully healed with the hard water constantly irritating my skin.

Travelling between the various properties was proof to me of how water affects skin. I had been looking at this previously and had seen changes but never put it down to water as specifically as I did when I travelled between Marbella, London and Lisbon.

A few hours drive from Lisbon, I sometimes go to a villa I own in the Algarve which also has the mother of all water softeners. In fact, I can't wait to drive from Lisbon to the Algarve because I know my skin will fix itself as soon as I get myself out of the Lisbon hard water area and into the softened water of my villa!

Sometimes some things are right there in front of your eyes but you don't see them. Water and its effects on Psoriasis was one of those things!

Let me give you another slightly different example:

A friend of my wife's, started developing very bad Multiple Sclerosis (MS), Asking her questions subsequently, it turned out it had started around the same time she moved to her new flat. No one could figure out why. The doctors said the usual, genes and bad luck etc. There was no explanation.

No explanation until I visited her and noticed her bedroom window in her new flat opened onto a massive electricity pylon, metres high and so close that you could HEAR the sound of electricity buzzing!

I theorised that since nothing else had changed and she was fine before (though she must have had the MS gene), then all things being equal, the electricity must have triggered something in her body and continued to trigger it. I did not know much about MS or electricity at that time - but I subsequently looked into it.

A study in Sweden aimed to evaluate the association between occupational exposure to EMFs and the risk of developing MS. The research did find an increased risk of MS among men exposed to high magnetic fields in their jobs, including electricity workers.
Reference: Flodin, U., Fredriksson, M., Axelson, O., Persson, B., & Hardell, L. 1994. "Background radiation,

electrical work, and some other exposures associated with multiple sclerosis risk of disease." Archives of Environmental Health.

I am not saying the electricity pylon caused her MS but it sure could have and it was one of those things staring her right in the eyes!


Let's come back to Psoriasis and water and the need for softened water.

I know you are going to moan that now you have to spend money and that this book is pointless because it doesn't give a cure and wants you to spend even more.

Well, you don't have to. I am just telling you something that WILL work extremely well for your Psoriasis and can even eliminate it.

The big one is Vitamin D3 supplementation. Next is the softened water. It doubles up your results on the road to elimination of Psoriasis.

Every person is different and no one can give you a 100% guarantee on anything. Even if one could get all the factors right about a patient, they can have weird thoughts at nights for example, which can affect their skin!
Anyone that guarantees you a total cure for your Psoriasis is a fool or someone that is not being honest.

From founding and running one of the world's best-known supplements companies to working on patients as a complimentary medicine practitioner, I can tell you that each person is his or her unique individual and they react differently to things.

However we are all human and some things WILL work universally for us. Green Tea pills will burn fat for everyone but if someone drinks a lot of green tea during the day, the pills will work to a lesser extent.

Soft water will reduce Psoriasis DEPENDING on the person and all the other complex factors behind their Psoriasis.

I am asking you to invest in a water softener and no I cannot give you a guarantee as to what percentage it will reduce your Psoriasis by, as I don't know you and your circumstances.

For example, if you drink a lot of alcohol (more later) then the water softener will not work for you as well as a teetotal person because, they (the teetotal person) will not be constantly exacerbating their Psoriasis.

Should you invest in a Water Softener if you have Psoriasis?

Depends. Get a water testing kit online from somewhere like Amazon and test your water to see how hard it is. They are cheap and accurate.

If you already live in a soft water area, then I can promise you that your Psoriasis would be worse had it not been for your location. So you are lucky.

If you live in a moderately hard or very hard water area, then you will 100% benefit from a water softener.

Even if you live in a soft water area, you will still benefit from a water softener, though if money or space are a barrier, you may not want to invest in one.

A water softener is a machine that takes salt in the form of block salt or mass salt and sits at the entrance of where the water comes into your individual property. It softens the water before it reaches your bath or shower.

The machine itself is around £400 and up to £1000, depending on the brand and size. The salt needs to be replaced regularly depending on the size of your property and water usage.

However, the investment in a water softener is VERY worthwhile if you have Psoriasis. It needs to be a proper one which takes block salt and large enough for your property.

Usually within days, you will see an improvement in your Psoriasis. Your scalp Psoriasis will get better too (more on scalp Psoriasis later).

Soft water is so important for Psoriasis sufferers that as you can see, it is Number 2 on the list.

Unlike Vitamin D, it costs much more as an initial investment and subsequently to buy the salt but what price can you put on health? And in reality, how much are you spending on Psoriasis potions and cures with no results?

I know some people are sticklers for science and I understand. Whilst complementary medicine is not scientific, it still works as testified by millions worldwide.

However there is scientific data on the hardness of water and skin problems including Psoriasis so I will devote a few paragraphs to this. Hopefully it will prove a water softener a worthy investment for you to make.

Water hardness is primarily due to the presence of calcium ions in water. Hard water contains higher levels of these ions, while soft water contains fewer.
The hardness of water can vary significantly between regions due to differing geological conditions, as per my own example of Marbella, London, Lisbon and the Algarve above.
In fact, prior to installing a water softener in London, the water was hard and my own skin much worse.

Hard water has been shown to be potentially irritating for those with sensitive skin conditions, including Psoriasis. A study published in the Journal of Investigative Dermatology found a positive correlation between water hardness and the prevalence of Eczema, another skin condition with symptoms similar to Psoriasis, in school children (Danby et al., 2011). We will talk about Eczema towards the end of the book.

Research suggests that hard water may affect the skin's natural barrier function. This is critical for people with Psoriasis, as their skin barrier is often already compromised. A study conducted by researchers at the University of Sheffield and published in The Journal of Investigative Dermatology (Proksch et al., 2008) showed that exposure to hard water can lead to increased skin pH levels, thereby impairing skin barrier function and exacerbating skin conditions like Psoriasis.

Hard water can interact with soaps and cleansers, creating a residue that may further irritate the skin (more later on why you should avoid certain types of shampoos, soaps). This scum, which is not easily rinsed away, could potentially worsen Psoriasis symptoms.

Soft water, lacking the high levels of calcium found in hard water, is gentler on the skin. This can potentially lead to reduced irritation and inflammation, which is essential for individuals with Psoriasis.

Soft water may help to preserve the skin's natural barrier function by maintaining a more neutral skin pH level. This could be instrumental in managing Psoriasis symptoms, as noted by the previously mentioned study from the University of Sheffield (Proksch et al., 2008).

Not that I am a huge fan of corticosteroid creams but, some research suggests that soft water may enhance the efficacy of topical treatments for Psoriasis. A study published in the British Journal of Dermatology (Danby et al., 2007) found that the use of a water softener improved the effectiveness of emollients and topical corticosteroids used in treating Eczema, a condition that shares several similarities with Psoriasis. I will talk more about this later because sometimes it may be advantageous to use topical steroid creams to get the skin to a reasonable state for the sun to reach it, for example.

For Psoriasis sufferers living in areas with hard water, investing in a water softening system could be a worthwhile consideration. These systems remove calcium ions from water, making it "softer" and potentially less irritating to sensitive skin.

References
Danby, S. G., Brown, K., Wigley, A. M., & Chittock, J. (2011). The Effect of Water Hardness on Surfactant Deposition after Washing and Subsequent Skin Irritation in Atopic Dermatitis Patients and Healthy Control Subjects. Journal of Investigative Dermatology, 131(1), 98-104.

Proksch, E., Nissen, H. P., Bremgartner, M., & Urquhart, C. (2008). Bathing in a magnesium-rich Dead Sea salt solution improves skin barrier function, enhances skin hydration, and reduces inflammation in atopic dry skin. International Journal of Dermatology, 47(2), 151-157.

Danby, S. G., Chittock, J., Brown, K., & Cork, M. J. (2007). The Effect of Water Hardness on Surfactant Deposition following Washing and Subsequent Skin Irritation in Atopic Dermatitis Patients and Healthy Control Subjects. British Journal of Dermatology, 157 (Suppl 1), 23-30.

It is up to you but if you are really suffering with Psoriasis and it is ruining your life, your confidence, your relationships and so on, please invest in a water softener that uses block salt ideally.

Don't get a cheap one and then say it didn't do anything. Don't get an industrial one either, which may be an unnecessary expense - unless you can afford it! Get a middle of the road solid water softener machine that is installed (by a plumber ideally) into your water system and uses block salt to soften the water.

You will NOT regret this decision, I promise you. I have purposefully given you the above 2 things first.

**Vitamin D and a water Softener will make a dramatic difference to your Psoriasis even if you change NOTHING ELSE.**

Changing "nothing else" is an important factor to consider because I am far too aware of how set in your ways you may be.

People don't change for the most part. As much as they want this or that, quite often they are unwilling to give up what they love for that change. You know smoking is bad for you, yet you smoke. You may even try and give it up for a while but then you go back to it.

Only when you have a heart attack, you take it seriously enough and it becomes enough of an inconvenience for you to do something about it! Even then, some people forget and they go back to smoking.

Psoriasis is the same. Most people who suffer with it, DO want it to go away but when you start telling them that there is no magic formula and that they may have to change some things, then they find reasons not to do anything about it.

If you have done the Vitamin D and water softener route and your Psoriasis is still bad enough for you to be concerned about and not happy about, then we move on to more in the arsenal against Psoriasis.

Please bear in mind that the list of things that can help Psoriasis is not exhaustive. The purpose of this book is to give you the ones that really work according to my experience. I could tell you according to science but we all know science has NOT cured Psoriasis, so this is one area where you shouldn't be all stiff about "I want science". Have an open mind.

Some treatments may work for some people but not all. The purpose of this book is not to leave you in limbo.

For example I could tell you to try Homeopathy which really does work for many conditions and "can" work for Psoriasis depending on your particular body and also depending on how good the Homeopath is in asking the right questions and having the right knowledge.

But I am not recommending Homeopathy here, even though I know it is a good alternative way of healing disease.

My purpose for this book is not to lead you down the garden path but to share with you a group of common remedies and lifestyle changes that will work for the majority of Psoriasis sufferers.

# Number 3: Vegetarian diet + Intermittent Fasting

We will go over what you should not eat a little bit further along in the book. I know that for most Psoriasis sufferers, changing their diet long-term is a no-no at worse and difficult at best. As much as it will help, I understand that many of you will not want to stop eating the things you love.

Fair enough. Life is about balance and some people don't want to live a life they find depressing because they can't eat what they want. However, this need to eat what you want should be balanced with how much Psoriasis is affecting your life. Is not eating what you want more depressing than having flaky skin? Depends, right?

Everyone is different. Some people have Psoriasis all over their body and they don't mind. They go out in shorts and a vest. Other people have a small patch and it is the end of the world and they lock themselves in their room for weeks.

Some people can easily not eat or drink certain things and for others, not eating their favourite foods is just an impossible thought and they rather have Psoriasis!

The reason why I have put a vegetarian diet PLUS Intermittent Fasting at number 3 is because after Vitamin D and softened water, this is the most powerful tool you have in tacking your Psoriasis - though not as easy to implement. It is however less costly!

Some people put this as number 1 in tackling Psoriasis but I prefer to give you the easier options first and only hit you with this if your Psoriasis is still problematic, long term and stubborn.

Unlike Vitamin D and a softened water which will help you and make you better immediately, the diet route may make you worse at first (unlikely for most) and takes longer to see results.

I say "may" because chances are that it won't but if you are very toxic, then starting to eat healthier may begin to throw a lot more toxins on to your skin.

So what should you do to start?

The idea is to replace as much meat, complex carbohydrates and sugars with as much vegetables and salads as you can.

I am not going to give you specific portions or recipes. Everyone should do their best and you try and do your best too. Don't go overboard immediately. Just do it bit by bit and start replacing as many meals as you can which contain meat, shellfish, fish, pasta, potatoes, dairy, grains and bread with salads and vegetables. Rice is OK for most Psoriasis sufferers but not all.

The only vegetables I suggest you stay away from are peppers, tomatoes, aubergines, eggplant and potatoes; foods from the Nightshade family.

Please don't come back at me with "Oh there's nothing left to eat then"! There are plenty of alternative foods left to eat.

Drink plenty of water and replace meat and carbs for vegetarian sources as above.

The key is starting slowly in moderation and not going so hardcore that you become fed up.

The change in diet is not forever. It is just until you get your Psoriasis under control because if it goes out of control again, then you know what to do to get it back under control.

The Intermittent Fasting is the second part of your Number 3 strategy for beating Psoriasis.

There is no doubt that when you don't eat, your Psoriasis gets better. Try it! Don't eat for 24 hours, just drink water and you will see that your skin gets better. If you have very thick lesions, you may not see a difference but for people with mild to moderate Psoriasis, not eating means healing!

So what does that tell you? It tells you that food, messes your skin up! If this isn't concrete proof that the cause of Psoriasis lies somewhere in your intestinal region, then I don't know what is!

The problematic organ can also be the liver for some people, but generally Psoriasis comes from the gut region and possibly encompassing the liver.

Stress also triggers Psoriasis, because stress affects the bits that are people's weaknesses.

People who have a weakness in their heads, get a headache when they get stressed. People who have spinal weakness, get a backache when stressed. People who have Psoriasis get affected on their skin when they get stressed but the epicentre of the problem is the gut.

At this point you may be asking yourself why am I not mentioning pre and pro-biotics if the problem is from the gut? Because I do not believe the "cure" is necessarily in pre or pro-biotics.

If you have an issue with cultures in your gut, pre and probiotics may certainly help. We will be talking about them a little bit later too.

For now, let's get back to Intermittent Fasting. If fasting heals Psoriasis, then Intermittent Fasting is the next best thing because it is a lot less challenging to do and a lot easier on your body.

By the way, if you want to do a long water fast WITH the supervision of a doctor, then your Psoriasis will basically disappear after a healing crisis (where it gets worse - more at the end).

The reason why I have not put this as number 1 on the list is that I doubt you will realistically do this or do it for long enough. Sometimes it needs to be repeated too if you have had Psoriasis for a long time.

Intermittent Fasting is where you eat all your food in a certain time period and you won't eat for the rest of the day. It sounds a lot worse than it is and I promise you that when you do it for a few days, it is really not that bad and becomes a habit pretty quickly. You just need to start and stick to it.

Some people can only do around 16 hours of not eating (in any 24 hours), some less, some more.

Generally, it is only after 12 hours that you really start seeing a difference in health - so not eating for 12 hours is not exactly a big deal. You need to aim for fasting for 14 or ideally up to 18 hours in one go in every 24 hours.

As bad as it sounds, it is really not that difficult if you, for example eat your last meal at 4 p.m. Then you can start eating at 10 a.m. the next day. For most people, this is doable. You can drink water during the fast.

Another option is to have your last meal at 6 p.m. and your first at 12 p.m. the next day. This is an 18 hour fast which is really good and will give you very good results, not only for your Psoriasis healing but for general health and weight loss too.

However if you can't go so long without food, you can go for a 16 hour fast. Have our last meal at 6 p.m. and your first at 10 a.m. the next day. Or your last at 4 p.m. and your first at 8 a.m. the next day.

When you do a 16 hour fast, after the first 12 hours, your body starts to heal itself for a full 4 hours. If you do an 18 hours fast, then every day, your body is healing itself for a full 6 hours. In a week, that is 42 hours of pure healing that your body would otherwise never do, if you are constantly snacking and eating.

And you know what? I bet you that if you have Psoriasis, you are constantly eating and snacking. Am I right?

I really understand that you may be skeptical and you may not want to give this point number 3 a good go. It is not easy. But believe me when I tell you that people's diets are 90% of the time the cause of their chronic diseases.

Try your best. Definitely start the intermittent fasting even if you fast for just 14 hours, giving you 2 hours of detoxification past the initial 12 hours. There is nothing wrong with having an empty stomach as long as you are not starving or out of energy. In fact, you will probably find you have more energy when doing this!

If you find Intermittent Fasting very hard to do daily, then do as many times as you can in a given week. Once a week, twice a week and so on. Some is better than none and you will see results, though it may take longer to see significant progress in the elimination of your Psoriasis especially if it is stubborn.

Psoriasis is a strange disease. It is like it has a mind of its own. Even when something seems to be working, it suddenly stops working well. There are a lot of things in play with Psoriasis and you need to get quite a few of them under control to see great results.

There is quite a bit of scientific evidence for Intermittent Fasting (IF) and possible healing of Psoriasis and general inflammatory conditions:

### 1. Reduction in Inflammation

Fasting periods have been shown to reduce markers of inflammation in the body. A study published in Cell in 2016 found that periodic fasting cycles can trigger anti-inflammatory responses in the body, reducing inflammatory markers (Cheng et al., 2016).

Given that Psoriasis is an inflammatory condition, the anti-inflammatory effects of IF might contribute to symptom alleviation.

Don't forget also that most religions have some sort of fasting in them. I wonder why!

## 2. Autophagy Stimulation

Autophagy is the body's way of cleaning out damaged cells, which can contribute to inflammation when they accumulate. Intermittent fasting has been suggested to activate autophagy, which might assist in reducing Psoriatic flare-ups. A study in the Journal of Dermatological Science in 2018 suggests that promoting autophagy can attenuate Psoriasis-like skin inflammation (Yang et al., 2018).

## 3. Improvement in Gut Health

Emerging evidence indicates a connection between gut health and Psoriasis. Intermittent Fasting can positively affect the gut microbiota, leading to a more balanced bacterial environment. A review in the Journal of Nutritional Biochemistry in 2017 highlighted that IF can beneficially modulate gut microbiota, which may in turn impact systemic inflammation (Patterson and Sears, 2017).

## 4. Reduction in Weight

Obesity is a risk factor for Psoriasis, and weight loss can reduce the severity of the condition. IF has been shown to be an effective weight loss strategy. A study in the journal JAMA Internal Medicine in 2016 showed that intermittent fasting contributed to a significant reduction in body weight (Trepanowski et al., 2017).

Reducing weight through IF may indirectly alleviate the severity of Psoriasis symptoms.

**What you CAN eat**

All vegetables and salads apart from Nightshades (tomatoes, potatoes, eggplant, aubergine, peppers).

All fruit apart from Citrus, banana and Strawberries, though I would say initially you should not have too much fruits if you can and especially if you have sugar/candida issues (more later).

Oily Fish: herring (bloater, kipper and hilsa are types of herring), pilchards, salmon, sardines, sprats, trout, mackerel. Fish like tuna is a big NO due to mercury levels and heavy metals. Heavy metals are another thing to look out for with Psoriasis.

Poultry.

Rice, though some people may want to stick to brown if their Psoriasis does not clear up fully.

Herbal teas.

Oils such as Olive oil.

Tofu and organic soya protein.

Millet, quinoa, buckwheat.

All legumes: lentils, peas.

Honey, maple syrup, palm sugar.

Cashew, almonds, macadamia - basically most nuts and seeds apart from Peanut (and anything that your diary tells you is problematic - more later),

Soy milk, almond milk, coconut milk, rice milk.

Chia, flax seeds.

An example of something you can have at night is a smoothie or a soup made with beetroot, carrot, pumpkin, legumes and sweet potato. Do remember you can freeze the foods you make and have them in the following weeks to make life easier!

# Other things which will help your Psoriasis

---

I have a big list of things for you that will help with your Psoriasis coming up in this chapter. We are not going to cover things which "may" help some Psoriasis sufferers. I have purposefully kept this book to the point, so you get the juicy things that work.

In this chapter, the various points coming up are in no particular order as opposed to the first chapter where number 1 is the most important thing to start with.

The reason why there is no order here is that some of these points work better for some people and others may not even apply to you. For example if you don't drink alcohol, then staying away from alcohol will not apply to you.

Try and do as many of the below as you can but you may find that by doing just points 1-3 in the first chapter, your Psoriasis is so much better or 100% healed that you do not even need to bother with the rest of the book. It all depends on the severity, causes and duration of your Psoriasis. If points 1-3 did the job, be happy and enjoy life!

**Seawater and sun**

There is no doubt that bathing in sea-water daily and then catching sun will eliminate Psoriasis for most people. How does it do that? Possibly by reducing the skin inflammation by as much as 100%. The only issue for most people is getting those two regularly.

If you can get yourself to live near the sea, where it is warm enough to swim all year round or at least be able to dip yourself in and then catch some sun afterwards, your Psoriasis for the most part will be a non-issue. If you are one of the rare group of people (very rare) where this doesn't work, then Intermittent Fasting and a vegetarian diet will help to bring you to a level where sea and sun will work for you too.

The only other issue some people have is that they have so much solid dry skin that the sun just doesn't ever reach the layer underneath to do the healing. This is where Intermittent Fasting comes in to reduce the thickness of the dry lesions over time.

**Sleep**

Have you ever slept more than "your" normal and found that your Psoriasis is a little bit (or a lot) better in the morning?
I say in the morning because as the day progresses and you start eating, getting stressed etc, your Psoriasis may get back to normal.

Sleep has been consistently linked to optimal immune function. During deep stages of sleep, the body produces immune-boosting substances, such as cytokines. A study published in the Journal of Experimental Medicine found that sleep enhances the functioning of T-cells, vital components of the immune system. T-cells are crucial in Psoriasis, as they mistakenly attack healthy skin cells in affected individuals, leading to inflammation.

Chronic inflammation is a hallmark of Psoriasis. Pro-inflammatory cytokines, like TNF-alpha and IL-6, are elevated in Psoriasis. Research in the European Journal of Physiology has demonstrated that sleep deprivation can increase levels of these inflammatory markers. Consequently, adequate sleep might help reduce systemic inflammation, potentially alleviating Psoriatic symptoms.

There are other scientific explanations as to why extra sleep can help heal Psoriasis.

The hypothalamus-pituitary-adrenal (HPA) axis plays a pivotal role in stress responses. Disruption in sleep patterns can activate the HPA axis, leading to the secretion of stress hormones like cortisol. Elevated cortisol can exacerbate Psoriasis. Ensuring adequate sleep helps in regulating the HPA axis and maintaining a balanced stress response.

Chronic conditions like Psoriasis can take a toll on mental health, leading to conditions like depression and anxiety. Poor sleep further exacerbates these psychological conditions. On the flip side, good sleep can improve mood, reduce anxiety, and enhance overall mental well-being, indirectly benefiting the course of Psoriasis.

During the initial deep stages of sleep, the body secretes growth hormone, a critical substance for tissue repair and regeneration. Given that Psoriasis is a skin condition, optimal skin repair during sleep can potentially facilitate the healing of Psoriatic plaques.

The skin's barrier function is vital to prevent excessive water loss and protect against external irritants and allergens. A study in the Journal of Investigative Dermatology showed that sleep deprivation could impair the skin barrier function. For Psoriasis sufferers, a robust skin barrier is crucial to prevent flare-ups.

The general consensus here is that extra sleep, more than your norm, helps the skin heal itself. Whatever the reason may not be that important as long as you agree that if you can manage to get a little bit more sleep, your Psoriasis will get better.

There are of course, tons of ways to improve your sleep and I really don't think this book has the scope for all of them.

I will just mention a few: Melatonin supplement is good for falling asleep, Rescue Remedy Night Time Spray, Valerian Supplement, Chamomile Tea, Magnesium supplement, Meditation, good sleep routines, no caffeine before sleep, no TV or iPad/tablet simulation before sleep, no eating before sleep and so on.

Remember, as the sun sets, your eyes will know it is time to wind down. If you bring bright tech in front of them, they think it's daylight again and get confused.

Ideal sleep times for adults are at least 8 hours and children 10 hrs.

**Do not pick your skin - file it down or moisturise it**

One of the issues as mentioned above is that for some people, Psoriasis produces such thick skin that no amount of lotions or sun reaches the layer underneath.

It is very important that if you are going to take sea and sun that you make sure the sun reaches your skin. You can try medication to reduce the thickness of your patchy, dry skin areas. Whatever that works to enable the sun to reach it.

Picking your skin is really bad for Psoriasis. If you can, you should file it down.

There are these home machines for getting rid of dry skin on your feet. They are around £20-£40. Get one of those with a soft sand-paper and gently sand down your dry skin. A good one is the School electronic foot filing machine. Do it gently and make sure you don't sand it too much for you to bleed. Then apply some corticosteroid cream for a few days daily.

Sanding down and some corticosteroid cream will bring down the thickness of your skin and then you can get some sun on it.

If you are not near a beach or exposed to high levels of sun, you can get your healing UV rays in a tanning salon. Personally I am not a fan of fake sun and think it can be dangerous, especially when you expose Psoriatic unhealthy skin to fake UV rays. However if your Psoriasis is bad and you want to bring it under control, then sometimes a bit of bad is good.

Sea-water is very salty and that salt also helps to soften dry skin. That's why seawater and sun is the ideal remedy for Psoriasis for most people.

I have known people from Britain with very bad Psoriasis that moved to countries like Spain, Greece or Portugal and their Psoriasis totally disappeared, especially in the summer months.

**Stress**

Without wanting to exaggerate, the 2 biggest reasons for disease are food and stress. If you can get your diet right and stress levels down, you will probably be a very healthy individual.

Obviously, you can't do much about your genes, however if you can manage your stress levels and eat the right foods, then you can avoid the bad genes being triggered or keep them in check.

One of the most consistent observations made by both researchers and clinicians alike is the relationship between stress and the exacerbation of Psoriasis symptoms.

The connection between stress and Psoriasis is bidirectional: Psoriasis can induce psychological stress, and stress can, in turn, exacerbate Psoriasis. As a Psoriasis sufferer, you will know this already! However if you wanted scientific proof of this, then it exists!

Reference: Evers, A. W., Verhoeven, E. W., Kraaimaat, F. W., de Jong, E. M., de Brouwer, S. J., Schalkwijk, J., ... & van de Kerkhof, P. C. 2010. "How stress gets under the skin: cortisol and stress reactivity in Psoriasis." The British Journal of Dermatology. This study underscores the cyclical relationship between stress and Psoriasis, suggesting that high-stress reactivity may exacerbate Psoriasis severity.

When a person is under stress, the body produces hormones such as cortisol. While these hormones are essential in managing short-term threats or challenges, chronic elevation can disrupt immune system functionality. You may want to consider an anti-cortisol supplement such as Conjugated Linoleic Acid (CLA). This is not essential but if you are a highly stressed individual, it may help with your Psoriasis.

Stress can result in dysregulation of the immune system, promoting inflammation. For individuals with Psoriasis, this can mean increased activity of immune cells that target the skin.

Reference: Dhabhar, F. S. 2014. "Effects of stress on immune function: the good, the bad, and the beautiful." Immunologic Research. This research elucidates how stress modulates immune responses, which can be particularly relevant in autoimmune conditions like Psoriasis.

Stress induces the release of certain molecules, like Substance P, which are more abundant in Psoriatic skin and can intensify inflammation. Substance P is a neuropeptide which is released from sensory nerve endings and is widely present in nerve fibres

Reference: Paus, R., Theoharides, T. C., & Arck, P. C. 2006. "Neuroimmunoendocrine circuitry of the 'brain-skin connection'." Trends in Immunology. This article highlights the intricate interplay between neurological and immune systems in skin health and disease.


Stress not only worsens Psoriasis but the visible manifestations of Psoriasis can also escalate stress, creating a vicious cycle. This highlights the importance of effective stress management techniques for Psoriasis patients. So it can be a chicken or egg scenario where stress makes Psoriasis worse and seeing your skin all inflamed and full of dryness and scales can make you more stressed!

Reference: Zachariae, R., Oster, H., Bjerring, P., & Kragballe, K. 1996. "Effects of psychologic intervention on Psoriasis: a preliminary report." Journal of the American Academy of Dermatology. This study indicates that psychological interventions, like stress management training, can lead to a reduction in Psoriasis severity.


The intertwining of stress and Psoriasis highlights the importance of a holistic approach to managing this skin condition. Addressing only the physical manifestations without considering the psychological component may prove insufficient. Adopting stress-reducing techniques, like mindfulness, meditation, and counselling, can complement traditional treatments, potentially offering you a more comprehensive strategy for managing your condition.

Understanding this connection offers an empowered stance - highlighting the significance of mental well-being in managing and potentially alleviating your symptoms.

Stress is not the sole cause of your Psoriasis but it can make it seriously worse and more long-lasting.

Some Effective Stress-Reduction Techniques:

Mindfulness is the practice of staying present and fully engaging with the current moment. Meditation, especially mindfulness meditation, can help ground you, reducing anxiety and stress.

Reference: Kabat-Zinn, J., Wheeler, E., Light, T., Skillings, A., Scharf, M. J., Cropley, T. G., ... & Bernhard, J. D. 1998. "Influence of a mindfulness meditation-based stress reduction intervention on rates of skin clearing in patients with moderate to severe Psoriasis undergoing phototherapy (UVB) and photochemotherapy (PUVA)." Psychosomatic Medicine.

Cognitive Behavioural Therapy (CBT) is a type of psychotherapy that helps you recognise and challenge negative thought patterns, making it effective for managing stress, anxiety, and depression.

Reference: Fortune, D. G., Richards, H. L., Griffiths, C. E. 2005. "Psychological factors in Psoriasis: consequences, mechanisms, and interventions." Dermatologic Clinics.

Physical activity is a natural stress-reliever. It boosts endorphin production, often dubbed "feel-good hormones", which can alleviate feelings of anxiety and depression. More on exercise later!

Reference: Sharma, A., Madaan, V., & Petty, F. D. 2006. "Exercise for mental health." Primary Care Companion to The Journal of Clinical Psychiatry.

Deep Breathing and Progressive Muscle Relaxation techniques help in activating the body's relaxation response. By focusing on breath or gradually tensing and then relaxing each muscle group, you can shift from the stress response to a state of relaxation.

Reference: Varvogli, L., & Darviri, C. 2011. "Stress management techniques: Evidence-based procedures that reduce stress and promote health." Health Science Journal.

Writing can be therapeutic. Putting your thoughts on paper helps in organising and processing emotions, offering a form of emotional release. Try it!

Reduce the intake of caffeine, nicotine, and certain medications. These stimulants can increase anxiety and stress levels, and potentially exacerbate skin conditions.

Reference: Zarić, M. M., Aracki-Trenkić, A., Trenkić, M., & Manojlović-Stojanoski, M. 2017. "Effect of caffeine on the expression of a major histo-compatibility complex Class II molecule and inflammatory cytokines in the rat skin tissue." Acta Veterinaria.

Join a Support Group, as connecting with others who have skin conditions can provide emotional support and a sense of community. Sharing experiences and coping techniques can be immensely therapeutic.

Reference: Magin, P., Adams, J., Heading, G., Pond, D., & Smith, W. 2009. "Experiences of appearance-related teasing and bullying in skin diseases and their psychological sequelae: Results of a qualitative study." Scandinavian Journal of Caring Sciences.

This connecting with others works with some people but actually stresses others out! Decide, according to your personality!

Everyone has a different level of stress and manages stress differently. Most people who suffer from Psoriasis actually don't manage stress very well. That should tell you something in itself!

One of the biggest causes or manifestations of stress is irritability and intolerance. These can come from deep inside, such as a toxic liver or from something as simple as not having eaten and being hungry or being too tired or having had too little sleep.

You can control things like the above. You can make sure you eat before you get hungry. You can make sure you eat more protein foods which keep you full for longer. You can make sure you sleep enough and are rested every day. You can make sure you don't get yourself too tired.

A sure sign of being too tired, apart from being irritable is aching feet. If you have aching feet, make sure you put them in some warm salty water for 20-30 minutes and give them a good rub. Then elevate them for a while.

The feet are the gateway to health. As a qualified Reflexologist and Zone Therapist of some 30+ years, I can tell you that your feet have a lot to do with your health, but that is for another book - though we will address it a bit towards the end.

For now, just know that if you give the top and bottom of your feet a good rub and concentrate on areas that hurt and put more pressure on them, you will be less stressed and more healthy. Ideally, this foot massage should be done by someone else for total relaxation!

Live & love the moment. Try to forget the pain of your past and don't think of future worries. Enjoy the moment.

If you are anxious or stressed say to yourself:

"I am safe. There is no danger".
The brain hears this and calms you. Try it!

**Water**

My observations have shown that Psoriasis sufferers as a whole do not drink enough pure water. Alternatively they drink too many things that get rid of water such as tea, coffee and natural diuretics like vitamin-c-rich foods and drinks. By water I mean pure drinking water and not flavoured water, juices, sodas etc
At its core, Psoriasis is an inflammatory condition, resulting from an overproduction of skin cells. When these cells reach the skin's surface and die, it causes raised, red

patches covered with silvery scales, often accompanied by dryness.

Water plays a multifaceted role in maintaining skin health:

The skin acts as a barrier, protecting the body from pathogens, radiation, and environmental toxins. Adequate hydration supports this barrier function, ensuring skin remains resilient and less permeable to harmful entities.

While it's essential to moisturise the skin externally with the right moisturisers (more later), internal hydration through water intake can help maintain skin's natural moisture balance.

Water helps in flushing out toxins, which might contribute to inflammation, through urine. Do not underestimate this flushing power of water because without it, toxins are staying IN your body!

Water also aids in circulating essential nutrients required for skin repair and regeneration.

Dehydration can exacerbate the dryness associated with Psoriasis, making the skin more prone to scaling and flaking. Proper hydration can help maintain skin elasticity and reduce dryness.
Reference: Rawlings, A. V. 2007. "Skin hydration and moisturisation." Cosmetics & Toiletries.
Inflammation Reduction: Some studies suggest that adequate water intake can help reduce overall bodily inflammation, which is central to Psoriasis.

Reference: Boschmann, M., Steiniger, J., Franke, G., Birkenfeld, A. L., Luft, F. C., & Jordan, J. 2007. "Water drinking induces thermogenesis through osmosensitive mechanisms." The Journal of Clinical Endocrinology & Metabolism. This study, while not directly related to Psoriasis, underscores the potential anti-inflammatory benefits of water intake.

Proper hydration assists the kidneys in flushing out toxins, which might indirectly benefit you. While concrete evidence connecting toxin buildup and Psoriasis is limited in scientific terms, supporting your body's natural detoxification systems can never be harmful. Alternative medicine practitioners are all too aware of the important role of kidneys in many functions including its connection to the eyes and colds/flu.

Reference: Jequier, E., & Constant, F. 2010. "Water as an essential nutrient: the physiological basis of hydration." European Journal of Clinical Nutrition. This paper touches upon the essential role of water in various bodily functions, including detoxification.

If you suffer from Psoriasis, you really don't have to go far to see the effects of water on your skin! Don't drink water for a few hours and see how your skin gets worse. Start drinking a lot more water and see how it gets better! Not very scientific I admit, but most things that work are not scientifically proven per se!

Anytime you are dehydrated, maybe such as when flying, you will see your Psoriasis getting worse. It goes without saying then that your Psoriasis will get better with water.

Water is an essential route out for toxins. You could be doing everything else right, but if you don't drink water, you may not be rid of your Psoriasis as quickly as possible.

I observe this with people who want to lose weight. They can do everything right but not see much results. As soon as they start drinking more water, the results double because water flushes out the fat circulating around the body.

If you want an exact amount, then aim for 4 glasses of water per 50 lbs of bodyweight. It is better to have half glasses more frequently. Remember that your kidneys are one of the main organs of elimination and they work with water. If you don't drink enough water, you are not going to get your kidneys to do the job they have been designed to do.

## No alcohol, smoking or drugs

Alcohol is at the top of the list of "inflamers" when it comes to Psoriasis. Even if one assumes that Psoriasis comes from the gut and by gut I mean the small and large intestine, the liver plays a role in Psoriasis. Alcohol affects the liver.

This is why for some people, liver detoxifiers like Dandelion, Milk Thistle, Burdock and Gentian work for their Psoriasis even if for a short time.

Alcohol is known to stimulate the immune system, which can exacerbate Psoriasis - which as we know is an autoimmune-related skin condition.

Psoriasis is associated with the hyperactivity of T cells, a type of white blood cell. Alcohol consumption can further stimulate these cells, worsening Psoriasis symptoms.
Reference: Farkas, A., & Kemeny, L. 2019. "Interplay of systemic immune responses and local wound healing in the pathogenesis of Psoriasis." Frontiers in Immunology.

Alcohol can reduce the effectiveness of Psoriasis medications, making it harder to control the disease.

Combining alcohol with certain Psoriasis treatments can increase the risk of side effects, especially with Methotrexate or Acitretin.
Reference: Smith, K. J., & Skelton, H. G. 2003. "Drug interactions in dermatology: what the dermatologist should know." Journal of the American Academy of Dermatology.

Alcohol is a diuretic, leading to increased urination and potential dehydration. Dehydrated skin can exacerbate Psoriasis symptoms, particularly dryness and flaking. We talked about water and the need for hydration already.
Reference: Pagnoni, A., Kligman, A. M., & Kollias, N. 2002. "The effect of hydration on the skin penetration of topically applied substances." International Journal of Cosmetic Science.

Alcoholic beverages are calorie-dense. Regular consumption can lead to weight gain, which is a known risk factor for Psoriasis and can make symptoms worse.

Smoking and poor diet are lifestyle factors often associated with regular alcohol consumption, both of which can exacerbate Psoriasis.
Reference: Setty, A. R., & Curhan, G. 2007. "Obesity, waist circumference, weight change, and the risk of Psoriasis in women: Nurses' Health Study II." Archives of Internal Medicine.

There's a well-documented link between stress and Psoriasis flare-ups. While some people consume alcohol to manage stress or anxiety, it can often have the opposite effect, increasing feelings of depression or anxiety and, in turn, worsening Psoriasis.
Reference: Connor, J. P., Haber, P. S., & Hall, W. D. 2016. "Alcohol use disorders." The Lancet.

So if you have tried many things and you still have Psoriasis and you like to drink alcohol, then I have bad news for you! You need to stop drinking. In addition to the above reasons, your liver also possibly can't take alcohol and it is being pushed over the edge.

The same goes for smoking and using drugs. These things toxify the liver and your whole system and your body doesn't know what to do and so it pours the toxins into your bloodstream and onto your skin.

It may be that points 1-3 in the first chapter will heal your Psoriasis. But if they don't 100% fix your Psoriasis and you like your alcohol, smoking and/or drugs, then you will need to give them up, even if for a short while to get your Psoriasis under control.

Don't give them up for life. Just give them up for a short period of time where you see an improvement in your Psoriasis and then at least you see that they are causing your Psoriasis to get worse. You can then make a further decision at that point.

**No Dairy foods AT ALL**

Dairy foods make Psoriasis worse for the MAJORITY of people. For many people they CAUSE Psoriasis! I have personally not come across anyone with Psoriasis that did not have a problem with dairy.

We are generally not meant to be drinking cow's milk and derivatives of it. Some people tolerate it but many don't and hence why you have so many cases of eczema, Psoriasis, rhinitis, constipation and Irritable Bowel Syndrome.

If points 1-3 of the first chapter have not fully brought your Psoriasis under control, then you need to stop all dairy products immediately.

The consumption of cow's milk and its by-products has been deeply embedded in many cultures for thousands of years. However, there's a growing debate surrounding the appropriateness of humans consuming milk beyond infancy, especially from another species. This debate becomes even more nuanced when discussing conditions like Psoriasis.

The ability to digest lactose, the sugar found in milk, beyond infancy is a relatively recent evolutionary adaptation. Lactose tolerance developed in populations that domesticated animals and relied on dairy for nutrition.

Even today, many adults globally are lactose intolerant, meaning they can't adequately digest lactose, leading to gastrointestinal symptoms. This prevalence suggests that widespread milk consumption is not a deep-seated evolutionary trait for humans.
Reference: Ingram, C. J. E., Mulcare, C. A., Itan, Y., Thomas, M. G., & Swallow, D. M. 2009. "Lactose digestion and the evolutionary genetics of lactase persistence." Human Genetics.

Some studies suggest that cow's milk and its by-products can trigger an inflammatory response in certain individuals. Given that Psoriasis is an inflammatory condition, any additional inflammatory triggers can potentially worsen the symptoms.

Dairy might also impact gut health. An imbalance in gut flora has been implicated in various inflammatory conditions, including Psoriasis.
Reference: Michalski, M. C., & Januel, C. 2006. "Does homogenization affect the human health properties of cow's milk?". Trends in Food Science & Technology.

While the exact triggers for Psoriasis vary from person to person, many people flare-ups after consuming dairy. I have seen this myself time and again.

These proteins found in milk play a role in triggering or exacerbating Psoriasis in sensitive individuals.

Insulin-Like Growth Factor (IGF): Dairy products stimulate the production of IGF-1, which might increase skin cell production and exacerbate Psoriasis.
Reference: Cordain, L., Lindeberg, S., Hurtado, M., Hill, K., Eaton, S. B., & Brand-Miller, J. 2002. "Acne vulgaris: A disease of Western civilization." Archives of Dermatology.

Going without dairy may sound like a big deal but in this day and age, it is not a big deal and in most modern countries, it is easily done. There are so many dairy alternatives these days. By the way, why do you think there are so many dairy alternatives?  Because many people can't handle dairy!

If you have Psoriasis and you want it to disappear, then you need to stop milk, cheese (VERY bad), yoghurt and butter. Anything that is or includes dairy, even a minute amount is a no-no. Eggs are also a no-no because for many, they are a big big allergen.

Many alternatives are just as tasty. There is almond milk, soya milk and oat milk which is even possibly good for Psoriasis. Oats are potentially good for Psoriasis both ingested and placed on the skin. Several creams use oats as their base material for healing the skin (more later).

We will talk more about what to eat to heal Psoriasis shortly.

For now, apart from alcohol, if there was one other thing that needs to be taken out of your system immediately is dairy. In fact, I would even bring a point 4 in the first chapter and have dairy products as point number 4. This is how bad they are for Psoriasis sufferers.

If you are a heavy dairy user, you may not have even given yourself a chance to see your skin without the effects of dairy. By this, I mean if you eat cheese and milk daily, no wonder you have red and inflamed skin. Try going without them for a few days and see how the redness disappears and how your skin gets better literally in front of your eyes.
Next on the list is another big one for Psoriasis that must be avoided - sorry!

**Wheat**

The 20th century marked a significant period for global agriculture, with the 1950s standing out as a transformative era for wheat production. The Green Revolution, which spanned the 1950s to the late 1960s, introduced high-yielding varieties of wheat. While these innovations boosted food production, some suggest a link between the hybridised wheat and contemporary health issues, including skin conditions like Psoriasis.

The Green Revolution was primarily aimed at addressing food shortages in developing countries. Dr. Norman Borlaug, known as the "father of the Green Revolution", developed semi-dwarf, high-yield, and disease-resistant wheat varieties, starting in the 1950s. These varieties were quickly adopted worldwide, leading to a substantial increase in global wheat production.

The newly developed wheat varieties were different not just in terms of yield but also in their genetic makeup. Modern wheat has been found to contain a higher amount of gluten, particularly the gliadin component, which is more immunoreactive.

Psoriasis is an autoimmune disorder where skin cells proliferate rapidly. Several factors contribute to its manifestation, and diet is frequently discussed in this context. The potential link between wheat consumption and Psoriasis primarily centres on gluten:

Gluten has been suggested to increase gut permeability, especially in susceptible individuals. An impaired gut barrier can lead to an immune response, which might exacerbate conditions like Psoriasis.

Some individuals can have an immune reaction to gluten, which can further lead to or exacerbate autoimmune conditions like Psoriasis.

A distinct rise in celiac disease and non-celiac gluten sensitivity has been documented in recent decades. While various factors are at play, the genetic changes in modern wheat are among the speculated contributors.

The 1950s wheat hybridisation has undeniably transformed global food production. However, its health implications, especially concerning skin conditions like Psoriasis, remain a topic of debate especially as far as most doctors are concerned.

References:
Dubin, H.J., & Brennan, J.P. (2009). Combating stem and leaf rust of wheat: Historical perspective, impacts, and lessons learned. IFPRI Discussion Paper 00910.

Van den Broeck, H. C., de Jong, H. C., Salentijn, E. M. J., Dekking, L., Bosch, D., Hamer, R. J., ... & Smulders, M. J. (2010). Presence of celiac disease epitopes in modern and old hexaploid wheat varieties: wheat breeding may have contributed to increased prevalence of celiac disease. Theoretical and Applied Genetics, 121(8), 1527-1539.

Fasano, A. (2012). Leaky gut and autoimmune diseases. Clinical reviews in allergy & immunology, 42(1), 71-78.

Biesiekierski, J. R. (2017). What is gluten?. Journal of gastroenterology and hepatology, 32, 78-81.

Catassi, C., & Fasano, A. (2008). Celiac disease. Current opinion in gastroenterology, 24(6), 687-691.

For most Psoriasis sufferers, wheat and gluten are big triggers for inflammation. Therefore, I strongly recommend you stop eating all wheat and gluten products until you get better.

Gluten can induce an inflammatory response in you, particularly if you have celiac disease, as just mentioned. Given that Psoriasis is an inflammatory condition, consuming gluten can potentially amplify this inflammation, exacerbating Psoriasis symptoms. In many people, wheat is a big cause of their Psoriasis.
Reference: Bhatia, B.K., et al. 2014. "Diet and Psoriasis, Part II: Celiac Disease and Role of a Gluten-Free Diet." Journal of the American Academy of Dermatology.

Some research suggests that gluten might increase intestinal permeability ("leaky gut"), allowing undigested food particles and toxins to enter the bloodstream. This could trigger an immune response, worsening autoimmune conditions like Psoriasis.
Reference: Fasano, A. 2012. "Leaky Gut and Autoimmune Diseases." Clinical Reviews in Allergy & Immunology.

Wheat is one of the main sources of gluten, a protein also found in barley, rye, and their derivatives. Products that typically contain them include:

Breads and pastries
Pasta and noodles
Cereals and granolas
Sauces and gravies (as thickeners)
Beers and malted beverages

Processed meats
Soups

Additionally, many processed foods may have hidden gluten sources, such as gravy, so it's essential to check ingredient labels.

While people with celiac disease must eliminate gluten due to an autoimmune response to it, others without this disease report improvements in various health conditions, including Psoriasis, after reducing or eliminating gluten from their diets. This phenomenon is referred to as non-celiac gluten sensitivity.
Reference: Molina-Infante, J., & Carroccio, A. 2017. "Suspected Nonceliac Gluten Sensitivity Confirmed in Few Patients After Gluten Challenge in Double-Blind, Placebo-Controlled Trials." Clinical Gastroenterology and Hepatology.

The problem is, we have gluten and wheat in so many foods and even when people exclude these foods, they go back to them within days. For most people, it is difficult to come off wheat. However you must do this to overcome Psoriasis.

If considering the elimination of gluten to manage Psoriasis, starting with a trial period of several weeks can be beneficial. During this time, you can monitor any changes in the severity and frequency of Psoriasis flare-ups. I can assure you that you will see a noticeable improvement.

Cutting out wheat and gluten-containing products can

result in deficiencies in essential nutrients like fibre, iron, calcium, and B vitamins unless properly managed. If you are not sure, then consult a dietician please.

Gluten-Free Doesn't Mean Healthy by the way! Simply switching to gluten-free processed foods won't necessarily yield health benefits. Some gluten-free products might contain high amounts of sugar, fat, and artificial additives. Always read the labels. High saturated fat foods are NOT good for Psoriasis either.

## Palmers Cocoa Butter Formula

As a whole, the skin needs to breathe. It should not be blocked by anything. It needs to be clear to breathe and to throw off toxins and waste. Skin is one of your organs of elimination. Your skin also absorbs things.

In an ideal scenario, you should not be putting anything on your skin apart from maybe some olive oil or pure vitamin E.

However, some people with Psoriasis have such dry skin that sometimes a temporary measure may outweigh the need to keep your skin clear. I will leave the decision to you but if you do want to use something whilst you get everything else in order, then I have a suggestion.

As I am sure you know, the skin health industry is worth billions. There are so many creams and lotions out there and if you have Psoriasis, chances are you have tried a fair few of them and I bet with no success!

At best, they give you a bit of relief but then they either do nothing, stop working or make your skin worse. Some of them have horrible colour or smell. The nice smelling ones are the worst for someone with sensitive skin due to the fragrances used.

Many of the creams don't do anything but many of them also make your skin worse by making it more dry and more flaky. It is embarrassing when you have skin falling off you!

I cannot write a book on Psoriasis without giving you some guidance on the moisturising aspect of your skin health. This book is a practical approach to things that work and everything I have put in it is what actually works. On that front, one of the things that works for Psoriasis is one particular cream.

Even if you say it does not get rid of Psoriasis (it doesn't) then it really helps and makes sure you have less scaly dry bits.

I am making it clear that I have absolutely no affiliation with this company and am not benefiting from mentioning them apart from benefiting you by giving you this guidance.

Palmer's make a cream/lotion called Cocoa Butter Formula with vitamin E. This is a VERY good product to put on your skin once, twice or several times a day, especially after bathing. It is best to put it on dry skin.

Palmers make other similar products such as a coconut oil one for example but ONLY this <u>Cocoa Butter</u> formula works for Psoriasis. In fact, I would say the coconut one, like many other creams, makes Psoriasis worse.

There is actually a fair bit of research on the benefits of cocoa butter for skin conditions like Psoriasis.

The main ingredient of the Palmer's Cocoa Butter Formula, cocoa butter, is a natural fat derived from the cocoa bean. It's known for its profound hydrating properties, making it especially useful for dry skin conditions.

Cocoa butter forms a protective barrier over the skin to hold in moisture, which is particularly beneficial for Psoriatic skin that tends to be dry and flaky.
Reference: Scapagnini, G., Davinelli, S., Di Renzo, L., De Lorenzo, A., Olarte, H. H., Micali, G., Cicero, A. F., & Gonzalez, S. 2014. "Cocoa bioactive compounds: significance and potential for the maintenance of skin health". Nutrients.

Psoriasis is an inflammatory skin condition. While the primary benefits of cocoa butter revolve around moisturising, there's some indication that it may have mild anti-inflammatory properties, offering soothing effects for inflamed skin.
Reference: Martín, M. Á., Goya, L., & Ramos, S. 2013. "Protective effects of tea, red wine and cocoa in diabetes.

Evidences from human studies." Food & Chemical Toxicology.

Palmer's Cocoa Butter Formula is enriched with vitamin E, a potent antioxidant known for its skin-healing properties. It helps promote skin regeneration, which can be particularly beneficial for Psoriasis patches that need healing.

The formula has been touted for its ability to reduce the appearance of scars, which can be of interest for you if you have post-inflammatory hyperpigmentation or other skin discolourations.
Reference: Keen, M. A., & Hassan, I. 2016. "Vitamin E in dermatology." Indian Dermatology Online Journal.

If you want to improve the appearance of your skin and you want a relatively cheap and easy to get cream, then try Palmer's Cocoa Butter formula from chemists, supermarkets or buy it online.

Another one that is good but nowhere near as strong as the Palmer's one is Aveeno Daily Moisturising Lotion. You can mix the two of them together for a bit better results than the Palmer's one by itself.

Oats, scientifically known as Avena Sativa, have a storied history not just in nutrition but also in skincare. From ancient civilisations to modern dermatological applications, oats have been cherished for their skin-soothing properties. For those with conditions like Psoriasis, oat-based products, such as those by Aveeno, can be a beacon of relief. Let's delve a little bit into the science behind the skincare benefits of oats, even though I believe Aveeno and oat-based products are not as good as Cocoa Butter.

When oats are finely milled and suspended in a liquid, they create a substance called colloidal oatmeal. This can act as a natural emollient, helping to soften and moisturise the skin, providing a barrier against dryness.

Oats contain a range of compounds like avenanthramides that are known for their antioxidant and anti-inflammatory properties. This can be especially beneficial in soothing the red, inflamed patches characteristic of Psoriasis.
Reference: Kurtz, E. S., & Wallo, W. 2007. "Colloidal oatmeal: history, chemistry and clinical properties." Journal of Drugs in Dermatology.

Aveeno has seemingly been at the forefront of integrating colloidal oatmeal into its products. Aveeno products, enriched with colloidal oatmeal, are said to help in restoring the skin's natural barrier. This is vital for Psoriasis sufferers, as compromised skin barriers can exacerbate the condition.
Reference: Li, J., & Yu, J. 2019. "Effectiveness and safety of Aveeno Soothing Bath Treatment in pediatric subjects with atopic dermatitis: a single-center, open-label study." Paediatric Dermatology.

Oats naturally help in balancing the skin's pH. An optimal pH can further aid in keeping skin irritants and pathogens at bay, as mentioned already.

Oats contain saponins, which have natural cleansing properties. This means that while moisturising the skin, oat-based products like Aveeno's can also help cleanse without stripping natural oils.

Reference: Reynertson, K. A., Garay, M., Nebus, J., Chon, S., Kaur, S., Mahmood, K., Kizoulis, M., & Southall, M. D. 2015. "Anti-inflammatory activities of colloidal oatmeal (Avena sativa) contribute to the effectiveness of oats in treatment of itch associated with dry, irritated skin." Journal of Drugs in Dermatology.

To conclude this section, try Cocoa Butter and ideally the Palmer's one as I know it works. Also try Aveeno and/or mix them together.

If you are using something else and it really works for you, then stick to it - and let me know!

Do remember that putting creams and lotions on your skin is not beneficial in the long term as Psoriasis is an internal problem.

**What not to eat**

This is a tricky one. I really don't want to make it complicated for you. There are certain things that are a no-no for Psoriasis sufferers but the list is very much dependant on the person.

There are so many things dictating what agrees with one person and what doesn't. It is a minefield and that is why you may read one book that makes sense but when you put it in practice, it doesn't work for you. Every person is different. The complex formula behind why you have Psoriasis is intertwined with personality, bloody type, genes, your history (antibiotics use for example), diseases you may have had (STDs for example), injuries, diet, exercise, candida, sweating, stress, what you come in contact with (mould for example) etc etc.

You may think you are the exception and you may be able to eat all the things I am going to mention with no bad effects - but I doubt that, IF you have Psoriasis.

The nightshade family is top of the list here:

The nightshade family, or Solanaceae, comprises a group of plants that include commonly consumed foods like tomatoes, potatoes, bell peppers, and eggplants. Over the years, there's been growing interest in the potential connection between nightshades and autoimmune conditions, particularly Psoriasis. But why might nightshades be problematic for Psoriasis sufferers? Let's delve into the scientific insights behind this hypothesis.

Nightshades contain naturally occurring compounds called alkaloids. The primary alkaloids in nightshades are solanine, nicotine, and capsaicin. Alkaloids are a defence mechanism for plants, protecting them from pests. However, for some individuals, these compounds can have inflammatory effects.

Found in potatoes, solanine can be difficult to digest for some individuals, leading to intestinal inflammation (Childers, N. F., & Margoles, M. S. 1993. "An apparent relation of nightshades (Solanaceae) to arthritis." Journal of Neurological and Orthopaedic Medical Surgery). While this study focused on arthritis, inflammation in the gut can indirectly exacerbate other inflammatory conditions, potentially including Psoriasis.

Research has consistently highlighted the link between gut health and autoimmune diseases. A compromised gut lining can result in increased intestinal permeability, often termed "leaky gut", mentioned already. This can lead to the entry of undigested food particles and other substances into the bloodstream, triggering an immune response.

A study in Frontiers in Immunology indicated that gut health is critical in autoimmune disorders, with dietary components influencing gut integrity (Mu, Q., Kirby, J., Reilly, C. M., & Luo, X. M. 2017. "Leaky Gut As a Danger Signal for Autoimmune Diseases." Frontiers in Immunology). While nightshades weren't specifically identified in this study as a culprit, any food that can cause gut inflammation in susceptible individuals could potentially contribute to conditions like Psoriasis.

Remember, even a small amount can set your Psoriasis recovery back by weeks.

While there's a paucity of direct scientific evidence linking nightshades to Psoriasis flare-ups, many anecdotal accounts suggest a potential connection. Many Psoriasis sufferers report symptom improvement upon eliminating nightshades from their diet. I have seen this myself. You eliminate dairy, wheat, red meat, alcohol and night-shades and the results are nothing short of miraculous.

Generally, nightshades are a no-no for most Psoriasis sufferers.

It goes without saying (but I will say it anyway) that ANYTHING artificial is a no-no also. As a general rule, anything that comes in a package and is processed is probably not good for your Psoriasis. Here, I am really referring more to the people with stubborn Psoriasis that Vitamin D and a water-softener has not wholly or substantially contained.

So, no sugar, no chocolates, no sweets, no cakes, no sodas, no candy, no popcorn (or corn, which is very bad for Psoriasis), no biscuits.

No red meat, no fish apart from oily fish. No wheat, no eggs, no dairy, no eggs, no gluten, no peanuts, no sugary fruits, no fruit juice, no soda, no fried foods, no shellfish. No grains. Some people are OK with Oats but especially at the beginning, it is better to avoid them.

For most people also, no caffeine and no strawberries, though generally most fruit should be avoided initially. If you find this difficult, then avoid citrus fruits for sure as well as bananas which are full of sugar.

Another thing you need to know is that the gut is very sensitive especially if you have Psoriasis. Much like a celiac for whom a tiny bit of gluten can set them off, a chronic Psoriasis sufferer with stubborn Psoriasis is very much affected by even the tiniest of the offending foods and their effects can last weeks!

If your Psoriasis is stubborn and you need to go the extra mile, then NO, that tiny slice of cake because it is your birthday is NOT a good idea. A little glass of champagne to celebrate your dog's 18th birthday is also NOT a good idea. You don't want to trigger a crisis internally and get your skin to start flaring up and your gut to start pouring things into the bloodstream. You want to be detoxifying as much as you can until you are happy with your skin.

I am sorry if it sounds harsh but believe me when I tell you it will all be worth it. You will be back to how you were meant to be when you were born and then if you want to pollute your system again, you can do it knowingly and knowing what will come out on your skin as a result.

For the most part, certain things are not good for Psoriasis sufferers, as mentioned above.

But you know, it's complicated! For example, people with "O" blood type may be OK with lamb but not ok with pork and beef.

People with candida may not be ok with rice but most other Psoriasis sufferers are OK with rice.

Generally I would say stay away from the above but more specifically take control yourself and write down what bothers you. For example, for most people if they eat bacon, they may get a few new Psoriasis patches the next day. For others, it can be a tomato and those new patches will stay there until you use some corticosteroid cream on them. For most Psoriasis sufferers new lesions sadly don't disappear by themselves.

A daily diary will guide YOU as to what you should not eat and what bothers "you". It may not guide you as to what you should eat but it would certainly guide you to what not to eat.

When I say "bother" you, it can be a new patch or lesion the next day or so, or it can be more imminent. Watch out for things like: itching, burping, reflux, sneezing, runny nose, tummy ache, gas, hiccups, yawning, tiredness, insomnia and other things that make you uncomfortable. They are your body's way of saying a particular food is not for you and they usually occur within minutes (apart from the insomnia!). A very common one is a blocked/runny nose when eating wheat. It is your body's way of saying DO NOT eat this!

In fact, your Psoriasis can be caused by something as simple as you constantly eating something that is just not meant to be eaten - by you. Something like tomatoes or oranges.

Some people drink orange juice and they get a tummy ache; or they go straight to the toilet and think that's great: "The orange juice worked for me to be regular, hurray"!

I would say the orange juice didn't agree with you and so your body flushed it straight out!

These are the sort of things you want to be looking out for. Anything which is a sign something does not agree with you.

In fact, citric foods are one of the ones that don't agree with many people who have Psoriasis. Orange juice, grapefruit juice, lemons and so on.

Eating bad food in a restaurant and getting diarrhoea can also set your Psoriasis back. Be careful what places you get your food from.

Proponents of the alkaline diet believe that maintaining a balanced pH level in the body can improve health and decrease the risk of chronic diseases, including skin conditions like Psoriasis.

While citric fruits like oranges and lemons are acidic in nature, they have an alkalising effect on the body. However, some individuals claim that consuming large amounts of these fruits can exacerbate Psoriasis symptoms.
Reference: Trivedi, M. K., & Mohan, T. R. R. 2013. "Impact of biofield treatment on spectroscopic and physicochemical properties of p-anisidine." Organic Chemistry.

Some Psoriasis sufferers report that certain foods or drinks, including those that are citric, act as triggers for their flare-ups. This could be due to individual food sensitivities or allergies. The reaction is real though and

hence why you need to keep an eye out and have a diary to
see a pattern of whether citrus is good or bad for you. As
for now, I would put it in the "bad" category for sure.

Citrus fruits are among the foods known to release
histamine, a compound that can cause inflammation. For
some people with Psoriasis, this histamine release can
worsen symptoms.
Reference: Maintz, L., & Novak, N. 2007. "Histamine and
histamine intolerance." The American Journal of Clinical
Nutrition.

Some medications used to treat Psoriasis can interact
with certain foods and drinks. For instance, citric foods
might affect the way these drugs work or increase the risk
of side effects. In either case, we are working our way here
to ideally NO medication for you, if you are determined and
persistent enough to follow the instructions in this book
through.

As a side note, some Psoriasis medications increase the
skin's sensitivity to sunlight. Citrus, particularly lime, can
further enhance this photosensitivity, leading to "lime
burns" or phytophotodermatitis.
Reference: Stratigos, A. J., & Katsambas, A. D. 2005.
"Optimal management of recalcitrant disorders: Psoriasis,
atopic dermatitis, and vitiligo." American Journal of Clinical
Dermatology.

While citrus fruits are typically considered anti-
inflammatory due to their high vitamin C and antioxidant
content, they might be problematic for some when
consumed in excess. Overconsumption could tip the

balance into an inflammatory state, potentially impacting Psoriasis.

Reference: Chong, P. W., Beah, Z. M., Grube, B., & Ried, K. 2018. "Effect of green tea and its polyphenols on gastrointestinal disorders: an integrative review." Molecular Nutrition & Food Research.


Psoriasis and Psoriatic Arthritis are in many cases caused by acids: red meat (uric acid), citric foods/drinks (citric acid) and dairy products (lactic acid). Eating and drinking them is constantly putting the body in a constant state of inflammation.


**Keeping a dairy**

Following on from the above, keeping a diary is one of the most important things you can do in your fight against Psoriasis. A diary reminds you of things you have forgotten and solidifies things you may suspect, because you will see a pattern.

For example I had a patient that had sleep apnea and had tried so many things to be rid of it. I told him to keep a diary as well as other things, but the diary proved that the biggest cause of his sleep apnea was when he ate past 5 o'clock in the evening.

We suspected many culprits and we did many things that worked for him but in the end his diary gave us the biggest clue as to why he gets sleep apnea and what it is that is making his life hell.

If you keep a diary, you may find that something like Kiwi may give you (and keep giving you) new lesions. It can be anything. Usually it is the things I mentioned above already such as the nightshade vegetables or ham, but it can be anything. Maybe a can of tuna!

Honestly, if there is something I have noticed with people in over 30+ years of working with them is that their complexity makes predicting the causes of their illnesses difficult BUT most chronic illnesses are almost always diet related and usually stem from what people love eating the most!
Even if you say disease is genetic or caused by stress, it is the genes and the stress that combine with bad foods or lack of certain good foods to cause the disease.

If the chronic problem seemingly does not come from diet, I can assure you that diet plays some role in it. For example you can have chronic back pain. Not related to diet, right?

For many, it is, because their diet is so inflammatory (full of sugar for example) that they can never get the inflammation in their back muscles down.
Please keep an accurate diary and write down everything you think can be relevant including anything you suspect may be causing your Psoriasis. For example, swimming in a

pool (chlorine) can worsen your Psoriasis. Remember, it can be ANYTHING, food, psychological or environmental.

I had a friend of mine that was suddenly going bald. It was so sudden and almost immediate that he just couldn't figure out why. He hadn't kept a diary as such but because he was my close friend, you could say I was his diary and was doing his observation for him.
You know what was the cause? He had started swimming in this particular pool and they used a lot of chlorine and somehow this was not agreeing with his scalp. He was losing his hair at a crazy rate. He stopped going there and his hair loss stopped!

Examples of things that come out of keeping a diary: Allergy to plastic bags! Allergy to coffee. Intolerance of many foods. Irritation from sweating!

A diary can point out so many things if you write everything down and then sit down to decipher. By everything, I mean "everything". Let me give you an example.

I had a client that had tinnitus. It had started a while back and no doctor could cure him. There were in fact many "possible" causes for his tinnitus and neither himself nor anyone he had been to, could definitively tell him what it was.

The possible causes identified by doctors were: stress and anxiety.

The possible causes identified by me were: tension, wrong pillow, neck pain, muscular issues, posture, vitamin deficiency, inner ear, dietary issues, lack of sleep, sleep apnea or an issue somewhere else in the body, affecting his meridians.

How on earth can you figure out what if any of the above without a diary?

I asked him to start writing down anything and everything, however minute. His diary started to look very full with lots of information. For example: tonight I ate XYZ at X time, I had a bath/shower, the water was cold/warm, I was tired (or I wasn't tired), I drank XYZ at X time, I snacked on XYZ, I slept on an X pillow, I slept well (or not), I slept mostly on my X side, I had this or that pain, I woke up with tinnitus on left/right side, it waste X% severity and so on.

After a few weeks, it was obvious that he was getting tinnitus when he would eat late, snore and get sleep apnea which would affect his brain oxygen levels. He basically would wake up with bad tinnitus whenever he got sleep apnea. He would get the worst sleep apnea when he was dehydrated or would have a late meal.

The solution was to ensure he didn't eat late, he didn't drink alcohol late, he didn't go to sleep dehydrated and for him to address his snoring and sleep apnea.

It was no easy feat to conquer some of his issues as they were complex and needed things like weight reduction, changes in diet, exercise and habits. However when he got these under control, his tinnitus gradually began to dissipate.

THIS is the value of a well documented diary! When you put everything in it, however seemingly irrelevant, then you can go back and look for clues and repeated patterns. They are almost always there if you have done a good job of putting everything down.

YOU are your own best doctor! You will know what works and what doesn't if you just pay attention and write things down.

**No Sugar**

Some alternative medicine practitioners believe that the cause of many diseases lies in the patient consuming excess sugar. The simplest one that can be observed is type 2 diabetes where doctors and complimentary medicine doctors both believe sugar is the biggest culprit.

Sugar is the new age disease creator and its effects can all too easily be seen. Look at any nation that consumes too much sugar, look at their people and look at their disease statistics.

Sugar is ubiquitous in our diets. From morning cereals to evening desserts, it's an ingredient that's hard to avoid. While sugar may add taste to our food, its health implications are not as sweet. High sugar consumption has been linked to a plethora of diseases, including skin problems. Notably, nations with elevated sugar intake often show high rates of certain ailments.

When you consume sugar, it swiftly enters your bloodstream, causing a spike in blood sugar levels. This prompts the pancreas to release insulin, a hormone that helps cells absorb glucose for energy. Consistent overconsumption overwhelms this system, leading to:

Insulin Resistance: Cells fail to respond effectively to insulin, making the pancreas work harder, producing even more insulin, which can lead to type 2 diabetes.

Inflammation: Sugar, particularly fructose, is believed to cause inflammation. Chronic inflammation is an underlying factor in several diseases, including heart disease, cancer, and skin disorders.

Fat Production: The liver metabolises sugar. Excessive sugar gets converted into fat, leading to fatty liver disease, obesity, and associated health problems.

High sugar intake can also impact the skin. Sugary foods with a high glycemic index can cause rapid spikes in blood sugar. This can:

Promotes Acne: High sugar diets can increase sebum production and inflammation, both of which can contribute to acne development.

Exacerbate Wrinkles: Sugar can interfere with elastin and collagen, proteins that keep the skin youthful and elastic.

Research consistently highlights the correlation between high sugar consumption and increased rates of certain diseases.

According to the World Health Organisation (WHO), global sugar consumption is on the rise, with many countries consuming over the recommended 10% of daily caloric intake from free sugars. Some, like the USA, consume more than double this recommended amount.

You don't even need stats! Look at the size of an average American vs someone from a low sugar-eating country.

A study in the journal Circulation noted that sugar-sweetened beverages are linked to over 180,000 deaths annually worldwide, with 72% due to diabetes, 25% from heart disease, and 3% from cancers. I am sure this is a low number by the way!

Nations with high sugar consumption like the USA, Mexico, and Brazil, consistently show elevated rates of obesity, type 2 diabetes, and heart disease. For instance, the International Diabetes Federation statistics highlight that these countries are among the top 10 for diabetes prevalence.

A report in the Journal of the Academy of Nutrition and Dietetics found a significant correlation between dietary glycemic index, glycemic load, and acne. Countries with diets high in processed and sugary foods often reported increased acne prevalence.

You can see sugar is not good for you generally. More specifically sugar is a direct cause, yes CAUSE of Psoriasis.

One of the primary physiological responses to Psoriasis is inflammation. Sugar, particularly in the form of fructose and glucose, has been known to promote inflammation in the body.
A study published in the American Journal of Clinical Nutrition found that consuming high levels of sugar, particularly fructose, leads to an increase in certain inflammatory markers, such as C-reactive protein (CRP). Elevated CRP levels have also been observed in Psoriasis patients.

There's evidence to suggest that insulin resistance, which can be exacerbated by high sugar diets, might be linked to the severity of Psoriasis.

A study in the Journal of the European Academy of Dermatology and Venereology found a significant association between insulin resistance and Psoriasis. The regular consumption of sugar-laden foods and beverages can contribute to insulin resistance, implying that reducing sugar could alleviate Psoriasis symptoms.

***Read again: Reducing sugar can ALLEVIATE Psoriasis Symptoms.***
Forget the theories; I have seen this myself with patients. Sugar causes and flames Psoriasis.

While large-scale controlled trials are limited, numerous anecdotal accounts from Psoriasis patients indicate improvement upon reducing or eliminating sugar from their diets - such as my own eyes and patient histories!

A 2018 review article in the journal Dermatology Therapies discussed the role of diet in managing Psoriasis. While direct evidence connecting sugar and Psoriasis remains limited, dietary modifications, including sugar reduction, were found to benefit some patients, especially those with obesity or metabolic syndrome.

Emerging evidence suggests that gut health plays a role in systemic inflammation and could influence autoimmune disorders like Psoriasis.

High sugar diets can alter gut microbiota composition, as per research published in the journal Gut Microbes. As gut health and its microbial balance play a potential role in systemic inflammation, there is a plausible link between sugar intake, gut health, and conditions like Psoriasis.

At this point you may be asking, what IS the cause of Psoriasis and WHICH one of the things I mention in this book are going to cure you?

The top 3 points in chapter one are going to seriously help and possibly alleviate your Psoriasis. But as I have mentioned a few times, Psoriasis is a complicated disease and it is not a case of one size fits all. For example, if your particular problem is with excess sugar and you do everything else in this book but you constantly keep feeding sugar to your body and increase the possible growth of candida and inflammation, then you cannot expect to be rid of Psoriasis without addressing your sugar issue.

Think of a burst pipe. You can do a lot of things to reduce or contain the damage it is causing; you can put a patch on it, you can even divert it. However, if you don't fix the burst in the first place, you would not have fully fixed the problem.

With certain people and in fact in the case of Psoriasis, with a LOT of them, sugar is one of the biggest causes of Psoriasis for the aforementioned reasons, especially because sugar causes inflammation. As long as you are addicted to sugar and you keep consuming it, you are flaming the inflammation!

Sugar is of course in the form of actual white or brown sugar but also in all the other forms it comes in, both over and covert:

Sugary snacks, sweets, candy, pastry, fizzy drinks, sugar hidden in food under disguises such as glucose, fructose, lactose and also in the form of fruit juices and actual fruit. Yes, fruit is full of sugar and if you have stubborn Psoriasis or a big case of candida, you will need to knock it on the head for a while until you get your Psoriasis in check.

Sugar substitutes are also a no-no because they send a false signal to the brain AND they contain ingredients which are harmful to the body. However, I would personally say they are OK while you are coming off sugar, to ease the pain!

Yeast products are not good for you as they feed candida.

What is candida and how does it affect Psoriasis?

While Candida exists naturally on our skin and in our gut, problems can arise when there's an overgrowth, which leads to candidiasis.

A study published in Mycopathologia demonstrated that Psoriasis patients had a higher prevalence of Candida in their bodies compared to those without Psoriasis. The study indicates that the yeast could potentially play a role in triggering or exacerbating Psoriasis symptoms.

The immune system's reaction to Candida overgrowth might play a role in the development or exacerbation of Psoriasis.
Research in the Journal of Clinical & Experimental Dermatology highlighted that the immune system's response to Candida Albicans (a specific strain of Candida) could potentially exacerbate skin conditions, including Psoriasis.

Emerging research supports the gut-skin axis theory, suggesting that gut health directly impacts skin health. An imbalance in gut flora, including Candida overgrowth, might affect skin conditions like Psoriasis.

A review in the World Journal of Dermatology discussed the potential link between gut microbiota and skin diseases. While the research is still in its infancy, there's growing evidence to support the hypothesis that Candida overgrowth in the gut could be linked to Psoriasis flare-ups.

Some individuals might develop antibodies against Candida, suggesting a potential immune response that could be linked to Psoriasis.

A study in the Journal of Medical Mycology found that individuals with Psoriasis often showed increased levels of anti-Candida antibodies. This indicates that their immune systems were reacting to the yeast, potentially triggering or worsening Psoriasis symptoms.

I have personally seen patients that have given up sugar altogether and been rid of their Psoriasis within a few weeks. Some of them had a big flare-up before it went the other way and the skin started to heal itself.

The biggest issue here is that individuals who do have this problem with sugar find it EXTREMELY difficult to give up sugar.

Sugar is like a drug for them and as soon as they stop consuming it, they get all sorts of issues including a worsening of their Psoriasis, headaches, flu-like symptoms and so on.

Giving up sugar for some is like giving up heroin!

The trick here is to do it slowly and incorporate it as a lifestyle change. Sugar is also very much linked to our taste buds, so you need to keep pleasing the body and maybe have some sugar replacements for a while until you get used to it but please do it slowly. Salt can act as a replacement for some people also!

The easiest way is to still have a bit of sugar in the morning so you don't shock the body too much but then reduce it later in the day and every day have less and less sugar.

Some people run on sugar so it can be difficult but believe me when I tell you that when you are sugar-free you will be healthier, with more energy, no brain fog, better eye sight and with potentially no Psoriasis.

Some people are hard-core and they can go cold turkey. If you can just give up sugar immediately with no side effects and you have stubborn Psoriasis that the first 3 points in the book didn't fully alleviate, then go for it.

**Stop snacking**

We are not built to be snacking all the time, especially if we are not at 100% health. You body has its own complex pharmacy and detoxification centre. Given the chance, you can make any medicine within your own body to get well and you can detoxify yourself of most toxic health issues.

One of the things that stops you from getting better is snacking. In line with what we discussed above about Intermittent Fasting, snacking is one of the reasons why the body does not heal itself. It is because you are not giving your digestive system the break to operate as it should and detoxify your systems. Some people basically never have an empty stomach! They even wake up at night to eat. That is crazy!

Let's say you have an early dinner. Your body digests and then starts thinking about using the rest of the free time to detoxify.

"Sorry body! You ain't detoxifying tonight because I am going to have some crisps and a bottle of wine at 11 p.m"!

ANY food or drink is considered as snacking apart from water. Whether you are Intermittent Fasting or planning on not ruining the detoxification process, you cannot put any food or drinks into your mouth.

Delving into the scientific side of things, there are definite reasons why snacking affects the correct functioning of your body.

The body has natural detoxification mechanisms, primarily facilitated by the liver, kidneys, and digestive system. When we eat, especially foods high in sugar or processed ingredients, the liver gets to work metabolising and detoxifying these substances.

According to a study in the Journal of Clinical Investigation, the liver has a circadian rhythm influenced by eating patterns. Constant snacking can disrupt this rhythm, potentially impairing optimal liver function and its detoxification processes.

Every time we eat, the body releases insulin. Constant snacking, especially on carbohydrate and sugar-rich foods, means frequent insulin spikes, which can lead to insulin resistance over time.

A study in the Journal of Translational Medicine highlighted that insulin resistance is associated with chronic inflammation, a cornerstone of Psoriasis. We come back to this chronic inflammation, time and again.

The gut-skin axis theory indicates that gut health directly influences skin health. Constant snacking, especially on processed or unhealthy foods, can disrupt gut flora balance.

A review in Frontiers in Microbiology discussed the potential link between gut microbiota and skin health. An imbalanced gut flora, potentially exacerbated by frequent snacking, could play a role in skin conditions like Psoriasis.

Autophagy, the body's process of cleaning out damaged cells and regenerating new ones, plays a role in skin health. It is believed that constant energy intake can hinder the autophagy process.

Research in the Journal of Dermatological Science suggested that autophagy mechanisms might play a protective role in skin conditions, including Psoriasis. Continuous snacking might impede the optimal functioning of autophagy, affecting skin repair.

Stopping snacking is very difficult for some people but if your Psoriasis is stubborn, then you need to stop snacking especially if you know in your heart that you are a big snacker.

In fact, the harder it is for you to stop snacking, the more likely it IS one of the causes of your Psoriasis. Stopping snacking and incorporating Intermittent Fasting as often as you can is one of the best things you can do to overcome Psoriasis.

By the way, constant eating is the cause of many diseases but maybeI will address that in another book!

## Keeping regular bowel movements

One of the common questions they ask you if you are seriously ill is whether you go to the toilet regularly, usually for a number two but not going for a number one can be problematic too!

Constipation is the cause of many diseases. Constipation, a common digestive issue characterised by infrequent bowel movements, hard stools, or difficulty passing stools, often goes dismissed as a mere inconvenience. However, its implications on health can be far-reaching, with potential ties to various diseases and conditions.

Diseases Linked to Constipation:

Haemorrhoids: Prolonged constipation can lead to haemorrhoids, which are swollen veins in the rectal area. Straining during bowel movements can exacerbate their presence, leading to itching, pain, and even bleeding.

Anal Fissures: Straining can also cause small tears around the anus called anal fissures. These are painful and can bleed during bowel movements.

Faecal Impaction: If left untreated, constipation can lead to faecal impaction, where the stool becomes hard and lodged in the intestine, necessitating medical intervention.

Colon Cancer: Some studies suggest that chronic constipation might be linked to an increased risk of colon cancer, though this connection remains a topic of ongoing research.

Urinary Disorders: Chronic constipation can lead to urinary incontinence or urinary tract infections as the impacted stool can press on the bladder, causing issues.

Rectal Prolapse: Straining can cause a small amount of the rectal lining to push out from the anal opening, a condition known as rectal prolapse.

Diverticulitis: Constipation can increase the risk of developing diverticular pockets in the colon, which can become infected and inflamed, a condition known as diverticulitis.

Dietary habits are directly linked to health, as mentioned earlier. Constipation is very much a problem you need to overcome if you have skin issues.

Combatting Constipation:

Increase Fibre Intake: Consuming a fibre-rich diet, incorporating fruits, vegetables, and whole grains, can add bulk and softness to stools.
Reference: Anderson, J. W., Baird, P., Davis, R. H., Ferreri, S., Knudtson, M., Koraym, A., ... & Williams, C. L. 2009. "Health benefits of dietary fibre." Nutrition Reviews.
Stay Hydrated: Drinking plenty of water ensures soft stools and facilitates easier bowel movements.

Regular Exercise: Physical activity enhances muscle activity in the intestines, promoting regular bowel movements.

Avoid Over-Reliance on Laxatives: While they can provide short-term relief, chronic use can make the intestines dependent on them, exacerbating the problem in the long run.

Set a Routine: Establishing a regular time, preferably after meals, to use the bathroom can train the body to have more predictable bowel movements. Everyone is different. Some people need to go straightaway in the mornings. The point here is that if you need to go, you should go ASAP.

Limit Dairy and Processed Foods: These can exacerbate constipation in some individuals. If constipation is an issue, consider reducing the intake of these foods. You already know that they affect (cause) Psoriasis in a big way. Red meat, cheese and bread are big culprits.

Probiotics: These beneficial bacteria can aid digestion and promote regular bowel movements (more shortly).

Reference: Dimidi, E., Christodoulides, S., Fragkos, K. C., Scott, S. M., & Whelan, K. 2014. "The effect of probiotics on functional constipation in adults: a systematic review and meta-analysis of randomized controlled trials." The American Journal of Clinical Nutrition.

Herbal Remedies: Some herbs, such as aloe vera and senna, have natural laxative properties.

The definition of constipation does differ depending on who you talk to. Some people think going every 3 days is normal! For our purposes, ideally you should go at least 2-3 times a day and empty a fair load off your bowels. This is especially so if you are eating healthily 2-3 times a day. However once is the minimum.

If this is not happening, then you are not having enough fibre, movement, water and/or exercise or you're eating too much meat, bread, cheese and rubbish.

So many people just don't get what it takes to be regular. Many others have weird toilet psychology and have just been trained wrong or think in strange ways about having to go to the toilet.

Some people can't go for this or that reason, such as other people being around or needing "their own" toilet! The list is too long!

Needless to say, if you have Psoriasis, you need to do whatever it takes to make sure you go at least once a day.

Some changes that are guaranteed to help you in addition to the above are:

Eating several of the following every day, spaced throughout the day: prunes, dates, apricots, mangos.
Helpful are also: apples, pears and for some people, oranges. Obviously these contain sugar so you need to balance constipation and how bad it is with the need to reduce sugars for healing Psoriasis.

Some people go straightaway when they have orange juice, though personally I think it is the orange juice actually not agreeing with them (as mentioned already), but who cares if it gets the job done! Obviously if you have Psoriasis and it is not going away, then citric juices are not the best.

Movement is very important. Some people can only go if they have walked a certain amount or exercised a certain amount. Things like the trampoline or running can help.

The thing most constipated people don't understand is that eating fibre needs to be a DAILY habit. It takes a while for it to work so you need to eat fibre regularly, exercise regularly, drink a fair amount of water and MOVE!

In addition, you need to stay away from things which block you up - top of the list being cheese, red meat and bread/ gluten.

Are people in cultures that squat (Asia) rather than sit on a toilet (Europe/ USA) more regular? I really don't know but I can tell you that sitting on a toilet is a relatively new thing introduced in the modern world.

There is evidence of less constipation in nations that squat but one can also put this down to their diet, which is more rich in fibre.

**Exercise**

We talk about exercise in various parts of this book, however it is worthwhile to give it its own section as it is an important part of the road to recovery when you have Psoriasis.

Exercise is great for its benefits in sweating, detoxing, circulation (blood and lymph), breathing, reducing stress and bringing you in contact with fresh air when you exercise outdoors.

The best exercise is swimming in ocean water with salt and in nature. The next best one is swimming in a creek or a lake.

Do remember that getting hot is generally not ideal for those with Psoriasis. This is why the above is preferred to other methods. However I am very much aware that only a tiny percentage of you reading this book are able to swim in the ocean as your main mean of regular exercise.

Psoriasis is fundamentally an inflammatory condition. Research indicates that regular exercise can produce anti-inflammatory effects in the body. This is achieved by reducing inflammatory markers, such as C-reactive protein and tumour necrosis factor-alpha, both of which are typically elevated in Psoriasis patients.

Obesity is a known risk factor for Psoriasis, and adipose tissue (fat) produces pro-inflammatory cytokines that can exacerbate Psoriasis. By helping to manage and reduce weight, exercise can indirectly lessen the severity of Psoriasis.

According to science, Psoriasis patients have a higher risk of cardiovascular diseases. Aerobic exercises, such as walking, running, and cycling, have been shown to improve cardiovascular health, thus potentially benefiting Psoriasis patients by managing these associated risks.

Psychological stress is a known trigger for Psoriasis flare-ups. Exercise promotes the release of endorphins, which are natural mood lifters. This can help reduce stress and, in turn, mitigate the frequency or severity of Psoriasis flare-ups.

Many Psoriasis patients report sleep disturbances. Regular physical activity can promote better sleep quality, which might aid in the overall management of the condition.

Moderate exercise has been shown to boost the immune system by promoting a healthy turnover of immune cells. Given that Psoriasis is an autoimmune condition, a regulated immune system can potentially modulate the severity of the disease.

Given the potential for skin irritation, it might be beneficial to choose exercises that minimise skin friction, such as the above swimming.

I have witnessed something myself over the last 30 years of dealing with various ailments. It is that people with Psoriasis generally don't do a lot of cardiovascular exercise. Make of that what you will!

If you do end up exercising in a gym or at home where you sweat and get hot, then ideally you should finish the exercise with a 5-10 minute cold shower to cool down.

References:
Gleeson, M., Bishop, N. C., Stensel, D. J., Lindley, M. R., Mastana, S. S., & Nimmo, M. A. (2011). The anti-inflammatory effects of exercise: mechanisms and implications for the prevention and treatment of disease. Nature Reviews Immunology, 11(9), 607-615. ↵

Carrascosa, J. M., Rocamora, V., Fernandez-Torres, R. M., Jimenez-Puya, R., Moreno, J. C., Coll-Puigserver, N., & Fonseca, E. (2014). Obesity and Psoriasis: inflammatory nature of obesity, relationship between Psoriasis and obesity, and therapeutic implications. Actas Dermo-Sifiliográficas (English Edition), 105(1), 31-44. ↵

Myers, J., Prakash, M., Froelicher, V., Do, D., Partington, S., & Atwood, J. E. (2002). Exercise capacity and mortality among men referred for exercise testing. New England Journal of Medicine, 346(11), 793-801. ↵

Slavich, G. M., & Irwin, M. R. (2014). From stress to inflammation and major depressive disorder: a social signal transduction theory of depression. Psychological bulletin, 140(3), 774. ↵

Passos, G. S., Poyares, D., Santana, M. G., Teixeira, A. A., Lira, F. S., Youngstedt, S. D., ... & de Mello, M. T. (2012). Exercise improves immune function, antidepressive response, and sleep quality in patients with chronic primary insomnia. Biomed research international, 2012. ↵

Nieman, D. C., & Wentz, L. M. (2019). The compelling link between physical activity and the body's defense system. Journal of Sport and Health Science, 8(3), 201-217. ↵

## Sweating

The body has several ways of detoxifying. Just as not going to the toilet for a number one or two is not good, not sweating is also not great if you have Psoriasis.

Sweating is one of those bodily functions that people often associate with exercise, heat, or embarrassment. But beyond its role in temperature regulation, sweating serves as an essential detoxification pathway for the body. Let's delve into the science of sweating as a detox mechanism and the potential diseases linked to a lack of sweating.

The human body has millions of sweat glands, primarily eccrine and apocrine. While these glands are involved in thermoregulation, they also facilitate the excretion of certain waste products.

Sweat helps eliminate heavy metals like mercury, lead, and cadmium from the body, along with various chemicals and toxins. Heavy metal toxicity is a contributor to Psoriasis. In fact, if you have metal fillings, you will want to replace them with white ones.
Reference: Genuis, S. J., Birkholz, D., Rodushkin, I., & Beesoon, S. 2011. "Blood, urine, and sweat (BUS) study: monitoring and elimination of bioaccumulated toxic elements." Archives of Environmental Contamination and Toxicology.

Sweat contains antimicrobial peptides, like dermcidin, that can combat harmful pathogens on the skin.
Reference: Schittek, B., Hipfel, R., Sauer, B., Bauer, J., Kalbacher, H., Stevanovic, S., ... & Garbe, C. 2001. "Dermcidin: a novel human antibiotic peptide secreted by sweat glands." Nature Immunology.

For those looking to harness the detoxifying power of sweating, consider these methods:

Exercise Regularly: Engaging in regular physical activity induces sweat, promoting toxin release.

Saunas and Steam Rooms: These can mimic the effects of exercise-induced sweating, aiding in detoxification.
Reference: Jezova, D., Kujanik, S., Vigas, M., Koska, J., & Kvetnansky, R. 1994. "Sex differences in endocrine response to hyperthermia in sauna." Acta Physiologica Scandinavica.

Actually I want to address sauna and steam rooms in a bit more detail because they have all the right ingredients to help you with the detoxification process. Again, they are not a necessary part of the essence of this book but they can certainly help with stubborn Psoriasis cases.

Saunas promote intense sweating, which can help in flushing out impurities and toxins from the skin. This process can reduce the buildup of skin cells and possibly decrease the thickness of Psoriasis plaques.

The increased perspiration can also help in hydrating the top layers of the skin, providing temporary relief from dryness associated with Psoriasis.
Reference: Sears, M. E., et al. 2012. "Arsenic, cadmium, lead, and mercury in sweat: a systematic review." Journal of Environmental and Public Health.

Saunas, by design, are calming environments that help in reducing stress and anxiety, which are known triggers for Psoriasis flare-ups. The heat soothes the body, promoting a sense of relaxation and well-being.

Saunas can stimulate the production of endorphins, the body's natural painkillers, providing relief from Psoriasis discomfort and uplifting mood.
Reference: Hannuksela, M., & Ellahham, S. 2001. "Benefits and risks of sauna bathing." The American Journal of Medicine.

The heat generated in saunas facilitates vasodilation, which is the widening of blood vessels. This results in improved blood circulation, helping to nourish the skin and potentially promote healing in Psoriatic patches.
Reference: Laukkanen, T., et al. 2018. "Sauna bathing and systemic inflammation." European Journal of Epidemiology.

There's evidence to suggest that regular sauna sessions can elevate the white blood cell count, enhancing the body's ability to fight infections and heal wounds, which could be beneficial in managing Psoriasis.
Reference: Crinnion, W. J. 2011. "Sauna as a valuable clinical tool for cardiovascular, autoimmune, toxicant-induced, and other chronic health problems." Alternative Medicine Review.

Coming back to sweating, staying hydrated is very important to make sure you sweating system is working effectively.

Drinking plenty of water supports sweat production, ensuring toxins are consistently flushed from the body.

Consuming spicy foods can promote sweating, thanks to the capsaicin in chilies.

Sweating, while often viewed merely as an inconvenience or a sign of a good workout, plays a crucial role in detoxification and overall health. Recognising the importance of sweating, and the potential implications of its absence, highlights the need to engage in activities that promote it. Whether you're hitting the gym, spending time in a sauna, or simply going for a brisk walk on a sunny day, remember that every drop of sweat carries with it a small measure of detoxification.

Some people believe so much in the power of sweating for keeping healthy that they consciously do not use an antiperspirant.

I don't know if that is such a great idea because you don't want to go round smelling bad either! But if you can, then don't use antiperspirants or don't use them when at home. Or try and use natural ones such as crystals, though for some people, they don't do much.

Not using a strong anti-perspirant deodorant is not a good idea for the majority of people as they work, socialise etc. The better alternative would be to consciously do things which make you sweat more, so you ensure more toxins are released regularly and for that, nothing beats exercise and a good sauna.

By the way, I will need to mention that what you put into your body affects your sweat and specifically how your sweat smells - or doesn't!

It's essential to understand that sweat, in its basic form, is virtually odourless. The characteristic smell associated with sweat emerges when it interacts with the bacteria on our skin. There are two main types of sweat glands: eccrine (all over the body) and apocrine (mostly in the armpit and groin areas). The latter tends to produce sweat that, when combined with bacteria, results in body odour.

Some people naturally produce less body odour due to genetic factors. For instance, many East Asians have a gene variation that results in dry earwax and reduced body odour.
Reference: Nakano, M., et al. 2009. "A strong association of axillary osmidrosis with the wet earwax type determined by genotyping of the ABCC11 gene." BMC Genetics.

A diet rich in fruits and vegetables can potentially reduce body odour. Plant-based foods often lead to more pleasant-smelling sweat, while certain foods like red meat and certain spices like Fenugreek can intensify the odour.
Reference: Havlíček, J., & Lenochová, P. 2006. "The effect of meat consumption on body odour attractiveness." Chemical Senses.

Consumption of red meat is often linked to stronger body odour. The body struggles to digest certain toxins present in meat, which then get expelled through sweat.

We have already talked about red meat and how it should be avoided if you have Psoriasis. It is just too heavy on the body. Later on when you have your Psoriasis under control, you can resume limited consumption - but not daily!

I am not a vegetarian and I personally believe for some people, they need to eat meat but I do respect that everyone has their own beliefs and opinions.

Foods loaded with garlic, curry, or other spices such as the aforementioned Fenugreek can not only make your mouth water but also lead to sweat that has a distinct odour.

Overconsumption of alcoholic beverages or caffeinated drinks can alter the smell of your sweat. They can stimulate sweat glands and potentially change the consistency and odour of sweat.

Reference: Rosing, R., et al. 1989. "Psychological stress and odour perception." Journal of Investigative Dermatology.

High in sodium and unhealthy fats, these foods can lead to more toxins in the body, which might be expelled via sweat, intensifying its odour.

Some medications can change the way your sweat smells. For instance, certain antidepressants are known to cause excessive sweating, which can alter the odour. Homeopathy, herbs and supplements can also change the smell of your sweat.

Menstrual cycles, pregnancy, and menopause can lead to changes in body odour due to hormonal fluctuations.

Conditions such as hyperhidrosis (excessive sweating) or infections can alter sweat production and its odour.

Tips for Fresher-Smelling Sweat

Stay Hydrated: Drinking plenty of water can dilute toxins in the body, potentially leading to less pungent sweat.

Maintain Good Hygiene: Regular showers, using a few drops of tea tree oil, and wearing breathable clothing can keep body odour at bay.

Choose Fresh Foods: As mentioned, a diet rich in fresh fruits and vegetables might result in a less intense sweat odour.

Whatever you put in your body will come out of your sweat. If you smoke cannabis, eat red meat, consume spices like Fenugreek, man you are going to STINK!

## Clothing

Clothing, a daily necessity for all of us, can become a source of irritation if not appropriately laundered and can definitely make Psoriasis worse.

Conventional detergents can contain a myriad of chemicals, some of which may act as irritants for sensitive skin. Switching to biodegradable alternatives can offer multiple benefits.

Biodegradable detergents typically contain fewer harsh chemicals, reducing the risk of skin irritation.

Alternatively, Sodium bicarbonate, commonly known as baking soda, can be a viable alternative for synthetic detergents.

Sodium bicarbonate is a mild alkaline compound that can effectively clean clothes without the chemical residues that might irritate the skin.

Studies have suggested that sodium bicarbonate has antibacterial properties, which can aid in eliminating bacteria from clothes.

As for drying your clothes, sunlight emits ultraviolet rays, which have natural disinfectant properties. UV radiation can eliminate many pathogens, ensuring clothes are not just visibly clean but also microbiologically clean.

The sun can naturally bleach and brighten whites, reducing the need for chemical whiteners that can linger on clothes and irritate the skin.

Sun-drying can also help in reducing common allergens, like dust mites, which can exacerbate skin conditions such as Psoriasis.

When you have Psoriasis, the choice of laundry detergent and drying methods can make a significant difference.

In addition, your choice of clothing can also impact Psoriasis. Where possible, you should opt for natural fibres such as cotton, silk, wool, modal, viscose and rayon. Do bear in mind that they may have been made using chemicals, so before wearing them for the first time after purchase, it may be an idea to wash and sun-dry them.

References:

Nicol, N. H., & Boguniewicz, M. (2008). Wet wrap therapy in moderate to severe atopic dermatitis. Immunology and Allergy Clinics, 28(3), 707-720.

Pritchard, M. (2000). Environmental benefits of domestic laundry: Influence of washing machine technology and the use of detergent and rinse conditioner. Journal of Cleaner Production, 8(1), 1-9.

Drake, D. (1997). Antibacterial activity of baking soda. Compendium of continuing education in dentistry. (Jamesburg, NJ: 1995), 18(21), S17-21.

Yoon, S. S., & Brandt, L. J. (2010). Treatment of refractory/recurrent C. difficile-associated disease by donated stool transplanted via colonoscopy: a case series of 12 patients. Journal of Clinical Gastroenterology, 44(8), 562-566.

Kowalski, W. J., Bahnfleth, W. P., & Whittam, T. S. (1998). Bactericidal effects of high airborne ozone concentrations on Escherichia coli and Staphylococcus aureus. Ozone: Science & Engineering, 20(3), 205-221.

Arlian, L. G., Neal, J. S., Morgan, M. S., Vyszenski-Moher, D. L., Rapp, C. M., & Alexander, A. K. (2001). Reducing

relative humidity is a practical way to control dust mites
and their allergens in homes in temperate climates. Journal
of Allergy and Clinical Immunology, 107(1), 99-104.

## Disease trade-offs

One of the things I have noticed with people is that they
often have a trade-off between several problems in their
body.

For example, Eczema + Asthma or Psoriasis + Rhinitis. It
is no coincidence that there is some sort of family of
diseases. Maybe it's the body's way of keeping healthy by
keeping an alternative signalling and toxic-removal channel
open.

For example, if you put too much corticosteroid cream
on your skin for your Psoriasis, you may find that your
Rhinitis is getting worse.

If you take too much corticosteroid sprays for your
Rhinitis, you may find that your Psoriasis is getting worse.

If you were to stick to the theory that alternative
medicine practitioners believe in, then these sort of
diseases are the body's way of expelling extra toxins out of
the body. If you suppress them too much, they still need to
come out another way - otherwise you are in real trouble!

It is only when you have cleared your body from within that you will start truly healing. Disease trade-offs exist in many different variations. You may get better with your Asthma, but your Eczema gets worse or vice versa.

The point is that you cannot suppress all the symptoms of all internal problems in your body. This is what doctors try and do when you go to them with a chronic condition that in terms of traditional medicine is not treatable.

You will be placed more often than not on some sort of corticosteroid regime, either orally or externally or both and chances are your dosage will go higher and higher with time, making it near impossible for you to come off them or turn back time!

You go into the doctors office demanding a "cure" and they give you the best they have. The fact is though, that every pill and cream can have a side effect, taking you down a slippery slope.

## How mouth-breathing can be a problem

This section of the book may not apply to you but I do feel it needs to be addressed as I have come across some Psoriasis sufferers that are mouth breathers.

Mouth breathing has many causes, particularly allergies, which are closely linked with Psoriasis.

Allergies are another immune response. Many people are allergic to food or airborne particles and they have a constant blocked nose; hence they breathe through their mouths.

We are not built to breathe through our mouths. It is an emergency mechanism but for many people, it is the norm as their noses are too blocked.

Mouth breathing becomes the norm at nights for many but if you are particularly unlucky, then you may be breathing through your mouth for many hours during the day also.

Nasal breathing has an advantage over mouth breathing when it comes to the production of nitric oxide, a molecule that plays several roles in bodily homeostasis.

According to a study in the American Journal of Respiratory Critical Care Medicine, the human sinuses produce nitric oxide during nasal breathing. This molecule helps improve blood oxygenation. Impaired blood oxygenation can affect cellular health and function, potentially impacting skin health and detoxification processes.

Adequate oxygen supply is vital for the body's detoxification processes, especially in organs like the liver. Research in the Journal of Hepatology shows that liver function, essential for detoxifying the blood, can be adversely affected by low oxygen conditions. Since mouth breathing can lead to reduced oxygen saturation levels, it can indirectly influence the liver's ability to detoxify.

Mouth breathing often results in a drier oral environment, which can influence the oral microbiome. A disrupted oral microbiome can have downstream effects on the gut and potentially on the skin.

A study in the Journal of Oral Microbiology highlighted the relationship between mouth breathing, dry mouth, and microbial imbalances. Another study in Frontiers in Microbiology linked oral microbiota imbalances to systemic inflammation, which can affect skin health.

If you are mouth breathing all the time, then you need to look at your diet and your environment. Two of the biggest culprits in a blocked nose and mouth breathing are dairy and wheat products, so you will want to switch from consuming them to alternatives. You may find this switch alone will do the trick.

You may also be allergic to certain foods, hence why the "diary" chapter of this book is of particular importance. You need to write a diary and see WHEN is it that you get a blocked nose. Is it after eating bread for example? Or the cause could be environmental - maybe you were in a room with an old carpet or old curtains full of dust.

Mouth breathing at nights is slightly different. Some of the causes can be the same as above, for example wheat and dairy, so they need to be addressed.

However a lot of mouth breathing at night is because you may be sleeping on down and feather pillows or just old pillows with a lot of house dust mite. Dry air, such as that in winter, caused by radiators is a big culprit.

You may have a dusty room or you may have allergens or triggers in your room. It can be anything: room spray, dust, feathers, perfume, old mattress, heaters, grass etc

Some people have musculoskeletal issues. I have known people who can breathe perfectly fine though their nose if they lay a certain way or to a certain side. Pay attention to this.

Eating too late or having issues which cause snoring are a big reason for night time mouth breathing. Have a look at some snoring and sleep apnea videos on Youtube and do the exercises they show you to strengthen your oral muscles.

If the cause of your night time mouth breathing is weakened oral muscles - and it is for many people - then snoring and sleep apnea exercises will help you and if you continue and persist with them, you will find that you will no longer be a mouth breather at night.

Like anything that is difficult to conquer and chronic, such as Psoriasis, PERSISTENCE is the key. Nothing long term is going to disappear easily and quickly because it is embedded and habit-formed.

The good news is that if you take out dairy and wheat products, then a lot of your mouth breathing will stop.

## Hot baths and showers

I have noticed that many Psoriasis sufferers have several things in common. One of these things is that Psoriasis sufferers have a tendency to like hot baths and showers. I am not saying all, but many. If you or a loved one is a Psoriasis sufferer and you are reading this and you know that you take colder showers, then that's fine! At least you are doing something right.

Generally though, Psoriasis is a "heat" problem. So eating hot foods (as in heat/hot and/or heat/spicy), drinking hot liquids (hot tea/coffee) and taking hot baths and showers will not help your Psoriasis. Hot things make inflammation worse.

I am sure you have seen that if you take a hot bath or shower, you come out with your skin lesions much more inflamed and red. The problem is, we often don't listen to our bodies or we are not experienced in looking out for and trusting the clues.

There is quite a lot of scientific evidence pointing at an exasperation of skin issues and bathing in hot water.

The skin has a natural lipid barrier that helps maintain its moisture balance and shield against external irritants. Hot water can strip away these essential oils. We have talked about this a bit already.

A study published in the Journal of Investigative Dermatology highlighted that excessive exposure to hot water reduces the skin's natural moisturising factors, leading to increased dryness and vulnerability to irritants.

By the way, I have not been giving you all these scientific references for many of the points raised to waste your or my own time! They are relevant actual scientific studies that have significance to what is being discussed.

If you thought that hot water may or may not affect your Psoriasis, well, here is it, scientifically proven that it DOES negatively impact your Psoriasis! Take heed!

Heat causes dilation of blood vessels, known as vasodilation. While this is a natural response, it can exacerbate redness and inflammation in the skin, especially problematic for Psoriasis sufferers.

Research in the British Journal of Dermatology emphasised that vasodilation induced by heat can exacerbate the inflammatory response, worsening conditions like Psoriasis.

Hot water can enhance the itching sensation, known as pruritus. For Psoriasis patients, itching is a common symptom, and hot baths or showers can magnify this discomfort. If you have Psoriasis and it does not itch, then you are lucky.

A study in the Journal of the American Academy of Dermatology revealed that hot water exposure can heighten the itching sensation, especially in individuals with underlying skin conditions.

Prolonged exposure to hot water can lead to dehydration of the skin's outer layers, leading to flakiness, tightness, and irritation.

A publication in the International Journal of Cosmetic Science discussed how hot water baths can accelerate transepidermal water loss (TEWL), resulting in dehydrated skin. This dehydration can exacerbate the scaling commonly seen in Psoriasis.

There's some evidence to suggest that heat shock can stimulate certain cells in the immune system, which could further aggravate conditions like Psoriasis.

Research in Immunity & Ageing discussed how heat shock proteins, activated by stressors like hot water, can influence the immune response. Given Psoriasis is an autoimmune condition, excessive activation of the immune response can potentially worsen the condition.

I know it is hard for some people to lower the temperature of their baths or showers. But you need to! You will get used to it, I promise. Just like how you've gotten used to hot baths, you can get used to cooler baths. Cold showers have also been shown to give you a better immune response which is so important when it comes to immune system issues such as Psoriasis.

Even if you have a warmer shower, finish it off with a quick burst of cold water.

Cold exposure, including cold showers, can stimulate the body's metabolic rate. This increase in metabolism can lead to a rise in white blood cell production, crucial soldiers of our immune system.

A study in the Journal of Clinical Immunology found that individuals exposed to cold temperatures had increased levels of certain types of immune cells. The reason? The body, in trying to warm itself, sees a spike in metabolic rate, which in turn can lead to increased white blood cell production.

Cold water can stimulate blood circulation, ensuring that nutrients and immune cells are effectively distributed throughout the body.

A publication in the North American Journal of Medical Sciences explained that cold exposure causes vasoconstriction - the narrowing of blood vessels - which upon rewarming, promotes vasodilation. This ebb and flow can lead to improved overall circulation.

Cold showers can be a form of acute stress on the body. Over time, regular exposure can make the body more resilient to stress, which in turn can benefit the immune system.

A study conducted in the PLOS One journal found that participants who took regular cold showers reported fewer sick days than those who didn't. While not directly linked to immune markers, the resilience to illness might suggest an indirect benefit to the immune system, possibly due to increased stress resilience.

Cold exposure activates brown fat, a type of fat tissue that generates heat and boosts metabolic rate. An active metabolic rate can, in turn, support a healthy immune system.

Research in the Journal of Endocrinology and Metabolism detailed the role of brown fat in metabolism and energy regulation. While the direct link to immunity is still being explored, the metabolic boost from brown fat activation may indirectly support immune function.

I am not saying for you to start taking cold showers, but it is an idea! At least sometimes!

## Mould

Whilst this may not apply to all of you with Psoriasis, it can apply to some. It may even apply to you but you may not know it because mould can be hidden in some foods, specifically peanuts and peanut butter or it can hidden in a part of your house that you may not see or notice.

As we have stated, while genetics play a pivotal role in the onset of Psoriasis, various environmental factors can act as triggers. Mould, commonly found in damp conditions both in food and homes, has recently been investigated for its potential association with Psoriasis.

Mould is a type of fungus that thrives in moist conditions. In the home, mould typically develops in damp areas like bathrooms, basements and around leaks. In food, mould can grow on products that are stored improperly or kept for too long. Sometimes you may buy a product that already has mould such as Peanut butter. While mould can produce harmful mycotoxins, it's the allergenic proteins that have sparked discussions around its connection to autoimmune conditions like Psoriasis.

Mould spores are known allergens. When inhaled or ingested, they can trigger an immune response in susceptible individuals. Chronic exposure to mould can cause a persistent immune response, which can exacerbate or even unleash conditions like Psoriasis.

Some moulds produce mycotoxins, which are toxic compounds. Research has shown that these mycotoxins can induce inflammation, a hallmark feature of Psoriasis.

Some epidemiological studies have noted a higher incidence of Psoriasis flare-ups in individuals living in damp, mouldy houses.

The consumption of mouldy food products, rich in mycotoxins, has been suggested as a potential trigger for Psoriasis in susceptible individuals.

References:
Bush, R. K., & Portnoy, J. M. (2001). The role and abatement of fungal allergens in allergic diseases. Journal of Allergy and Clinical Immunology, 107(3), S430-S440.

Islam, Z., Gray, J. S., & Pestka, J. J. (2006). p38 Mitogen-activated protein kinase mediates IL-8 induction by the ribotoxin deoxynivalenol in human monocytes. Toxicology and applied pharmacology, 213(3), 235-244.

Ma, Y. C., Lin, C. C., & Yang, S. Y. (2019). Prevalence and risk factors for self-reported skin diseases, skin-related symptoms, and impaired quality of life in rural communities. Journal of the Formosan Medical Association, 118(4), 805-814.

Wawruszak, A., Czerwonka, A., Okła, K., & Rzeski, W. (2015). Antifungal activity of the synthetic peptide LTX-315 towards Malassezia furfur, Malassezia sympodialis, and Malassezia globosa. Acta Biochimica Polonica, 62(4), 845-849.

If you see mould in food or suspect it, then do not eat that food. If you have mould in your house, you need to treat it.

**What shampoo to use**

One of the biggest issues for people with Psoriasis is scalp issues and scalp Psoriasis. In fact, for many, it is a bigger issue that the rest of their body, because they can hide the rest of their body.

Psoriasis can cause unsightly scaling and dandruff and psychologically affect someone to a great extent especially when the scalp and hair are affected. Psoriasis can also cause hair loss.

Obviously the general methods mentioned in this book especially the ones mentioned earlier will be of great help to the overall treatment of Psoriasis.

However, have you thought why the scalp is so badly affected? Could it be something to do with what you put on it regularly? Something like a chemical-ladened thing called a shampoo?!

It is no exaggeration to tell you that I have seen people with horrific scalp Psoriasis go to NO Psoriasis on the scalp by just switching shampoos.

Whatever shampoo they were using was causing a lot of problems with their skin. Some people used the same shampoo every day, others used different ones but what they all had in common was that these shampoos were not natural and with as little chemicals as possible. They were full of SLS and SLES.

***When you have Psoriasis, you want to use a gentle shampoo with no harmful Sulfates such as Sodium Lauryl or Sodium Laureth .***

Sodium Laureth Sulfate (SLES) is a commonly used detergent and surfactant found in many personal care products such as shampoos, body washes, and toothpaste. While this ingredient is popular for its ability to produce a rich lather, its origins and potential to irritate the skin are lesser-known.

Origin as a Skin Irritant in Warfare!

There is a common theory that SLES was developed during wartime as a skin irritant. In truth, there is no strong historical or scientific evidence to suggest that SLES was intentionally developed or used as a weapon in war. This narrative might have stemmed from the potential of detergents and surfactants to irritate the skin, but this is not exclusive to SLES nor was it purposefully manufactured for this use in conflict scenarios.

However, it is true that some individuals find SLES to be irritating to the skin. The mechanism lies in its potential to strip the skin of its natural oils, disrupting the skin's natural barrier. This disruption can leave the skin vulnerable to external aggressors and can trigger or exacerbate skin conditions like eczema and Psoriasis.

Eczema: A study conducted by Ebling in 1992 showed that detergents, including SLES, can exacerbate eczema in predisposed individuals by aggravating skin dryness and interrupting the skin's natural barrier (Ebling, F. J. G. 1992. "Eczema and Dry Skin in Adolescents: Prevalence, Incidence and Variability." Paediatric Dermatology, 9(1): 8-12.).

A study by Neumann and Shemer (2000) found that surfactants like SLES can be irritants, which may lead to worsening of Psoriasis in some individuals (Neumann, H. A. M., & Shemer, A. 2000. "Environmental factors and Psoriasis." Clinical Dermatology, 18(5): 589-594.).

Many shampoo manufacturers call their shampoo "herbal" and add a whole load of unnecessary oils and herbs and THEY can also become irritants for the scalp.

The best shampoo you can buy for your Psoriasis is a simple one with ideally 1-2% Zinc Pyrithione. Look in the ingredients section and make sure you don't see the words Sodium Lauryl or Sodium Laureth. In the USA, Zeal is a very good shampoo for Psoriasis - and no I am not getting a kickback from them! Just telling you something that works.

Stay away from any extra herbs and potions. Companies add a lot of  ingredients that are buzz words to their products (aloe, caffeine, cannabis, collagen) for the sake of label claims. They are potentially (and often are) harmful to the sensitive scalp of someone with Psoriasis.

Not washing your hair is not clever either because you don't want a build-up of oils, allergens and dirt.

You will want to use softened water on your hair and wash it once every 1-2 days with a simple shampoo as above. Do not put anything else on your hair after washing. No hair gel, hair spray, hair thickeners, colours, no powders and no other artificial stuff.

Occasionally, especially if you have done something that has caused a flare-up and whilst you are adjusting your diet and doing everything else in this book, you may want to apply a thin layer of corticosteroid cream/lotion to an area of your scalp that has a flare-up.

However, generally, if you have got everything else in this book under control and you are not intentionally (or unintentionally) using an irritant on your scalp, then your scalp will also follow suit and heal.

## Chemicals on your skin

Following on from the above, it is a logical progression to talk about chemicals on your skin.

Your skin is a living and breathing organ and needs to "breathe". It needs fresh air and needs to not be blocked.

These days it is so scary to see sponsored Youtube videos selling "skincare" products to pre-teens. The word "care" is a very deceptive one when it comes to the skin and the products being sold for its care.

Walk into the beauty section of any mall and you see kids as young as 8 years old looking at beauty and skincare products!

Society is moving in a direction that is not healthy. However, even before now and the sale of harmful products to pre-teens, people have been using products on their skin that is not necessarily good for them.

Everyone is different, however a person that has Psoriasis should see themselves as different from others and should not follow the trends that others follow, as much as you may want to.

A Psoriasis sufferer is generally more sensitive personally, emotionally and dermatologically!

It goes without saying that you should not be putting any creams, gels, sprays, fragrance, oils, portions or lotions on your skin. The only thing I would personally recommend is olive oil, vitamin E and the Palmer's Cocoa Butter Formula mentioned earlier.

The skincare industry is worth billions and the Psoriasis and Eczema skincare industry worth millions.

***Psoriasis for the most part is an internal problem and no amount of outside creams will "fix it". Remember this!***

The skincare industry continues to thrive with a diverse array of products catering to various skin types and conditions. However, the same creams and lotions that can be adored by many, can be detrimental for those with certain skin conditions like Psoriasis.

The skin of Psoriasis patients is inherently compromised. According to The Journal of Clinical and Aesthetic Dermatology, the skin barrier of Psoriasis sufferers can be disrupted, making it more permeable and less capable of retaining moisture (Proksch, E., Brandner, J. M., & Jensen, J. M. 2008. "The skin: an indispensable barrier." The Journal of Clinical and Aesthetic Dermatology, 1(6): 22-31). As a result, Psoriatic skin is more vulnerable to external irritants.

One of the most common culprits in skincare products is added fragrance. A study published in the American Journal of Clinical Dermatology showed that fragrances are among the top five allergens leading to skin reactions (Johansen, J. D. 2003. "Fragrance contact allergy: a clinical review." American Journal of Clinical Dermatology, 4(11): 789-798). For Psoriasis sufferers, this can lead to further inflammation and exacerbation of their condition.

Often found in toners, cleansers, and some creams, alcohol can be drying and irritating for Psoriatic skin. Its drying effects can disrupt the already fragile skin barrier, making Psoriasis symptoms more pronounced.

Parabens, methylisothiazolinone, and formaldehyde releasers are common preservatives in skincare products. Some studies, like those presented in the journal Contact Dermatitis, have linked these ingredients to skin reactions and irritations (Bruze, M. 2000. "Preservatives in cosmetics." Contact Dermatitis, 42(3): 130-134).

We have mentioned this already but Sodium Laureth Sulfate (SLES) and its counterparts found in cleansers can strip the skin of its natural oils. For Psoriasis sufferers, this can lead to worsening dryness and irritation.

Many over-the-counter products promote the benefits of exfoliation, and while this can be beneficial for many skin types, aggressive exfoliation can be harmful to Psoriatic skin. Over-exfoliating can lead to increased inflammation and potential injury, further exacerbating Psoriasis symptoms.

The biggest external thing you can do for yourself is to get a water softener machine installed in your home. This is worth more than any potion you can buy that promise the world.

**Foods that are actually good for Psoriasis**

Your diary will definitely tell you what foods are bad for Psoriasis because they will make your skin worse and you will be able to literally see your skin more inflamed or new lesions appearing.

It is somewhat more difficult to know what are the good foods you should be eating to beat Psoriasis.

As aforementioned, the perfect anti-Psoriasis diet is one with no animal products, no junk, no sugar, no alcohol or drugs, no peanut, no dairy, no wheat and lots of vegetables and salads but nothing from the Nightshade family.

There are several foods including Fish you can eat which have scientific studies behind them and their potential benefit for Psoriasis.

**1. Fatty Fish and Omega-3 Fatty Acids**
Omega-3 fatty acids, commonly found in fatty fish like salmon, mackerel, sardines, and trout, have potent anti-

inflammatory properties. These properties can help reduce the inflammation associated with Psoriasis.

Reference: Gisondi, P., Barba, E., Girolomoni, G. 2018. "Dietary recommendations for patients with Psoriasis: Review." Clinical Nutrition. This study points out the benefits of omega-3 fatty acids in reducing Psoriatic symptoms.

## 2. Olive Oil

Rich in antioxidants and anti-inflammatory properties, olive oil, especially extra-virgin olive oil, can be beneficial for Psoriatic skin both when consumed and applied topically.

Reference: Ricceri, F., Pescitelli, L., & Tripo, L. 2015. "Diet in dermatology: Revisited." Indian Journal of Dermatology. The study mentioned the benefits of the Mediterranean diet, of which olive oil is a significant component, for Psoriatic patients.

## 3. Antioxidant-Rich Fruits and Vegetables

Foods like blueberries, cherries, kale, and spinach, which are high in antioxidants, can help reduce inflammation and the oxidative stress that can exacerbate Psoriasis.

Reference: Barrea, L., Balato, N., Di Somma, C., Macchia, P. E., Napolitano, M., Savanelli, M. C., ... & Colao, A. 2015. "Nutrition and Psoriasis: is there any association between the severity of the disease and adherence to the Mediterranean diet?." Journal of Translational Medicine. The study highlights the role of antioxidants in the management of Psoriasis and emphasises the Mediterranean diet.

### 4. Turmeric

This yellow spice, commonly used in curries, contains curcumin, an active compound known for its anti-inflammatory and antioxidant properties. Some studies suggest that turmeric might reduce Psoriasis flare-ups.

Reference: Antiga, E., Bonciolini, V., Volpi, W., Del Bianco, E., & Caproni, M. 2015. "Oral Curcumin (Meriva) Is Effective as an Adjuvant Treatment and Is Able to Reduce IL-22 Serum Levels in Patients with Psoriasis Vulgaris." BioMed Research International.

We will talk about turmeric and curcumin in more detail shortly.

### 5. Probiotics

Probiotics, found in yoghurt and fermented foods like sauerkraut and kimchi, can promote gut health. Given the emerging understanding of the connection between gut health and inflammatory conditions, maintaining a healthy gut microbiome may aid in managing Psoriasis.

Reference: Sikora, M., Stec, A., Chrabaszcz, M., Waskiel, A., Olszewska, M., & Rudnicka, L. 2020. "Gut Microbiome in Psoriasis: An Updated Review." Pathogens. This study underscores the relationship between gut microbiota imbalances and Psoriasis.

Some probiotics and probiotics come in Yoghurts and obviously if you are going to stick to the principles of this book, then dairy products are a no-no. You will need to find dairy-free alternatives. We will come back to probiotics again shortly towards the end of the book.

For protein, Tofu is a good choice. For carbohydrates, many people who have Psoriasis are OK with rice. I would say white rice is OK to begin with as brown rice can be heavy and difficult to cook, digest or find, if you dine out. Some people eat half and half of each.

Getting rid of Psoriasis which is stubborn may require a bit more effort. The initial methods in this book will greatly help but if you are severely toxic internally, then you may need to go the extra step to take yourself back to a good equilibrium.

If the above is the case, then yes, you will need to go that extra step and be more thorough. This means, organic over normal, brown rice over white rice and avoiding ANY foods that your diary has shown to trigger your Psoriasis.

## Psychological profile

Your mind and your psychological state play a great role in the fact that you have Psoriasis. The most obvious thing to point out here is stress. However, we are talking about a bigger psychological profile. Your general being, your mind, the way you see the world, the way you think, the way you talk to yourself internally and even externally, the way you view yourself, the way you walk and hold your posture, the way you see yourself in the mirror, all affect your Psoriasis.

The way you say "I am healthy, I am healing" vs "I have Psoriasis, it is getting worse" will have a direct effect on your Psoriasis.

The connection between the mind and body has been a topic of intrigue and study for centuries. One of the most fascinating manifestations of this interplay can be observed in individuals with Dissociative Identity Disorder (DID), formerly known as multiple personality disorder. DID is characterised by the presence of two or more distinct personality states that control an individual's behaviour, consciousness, and memory.

There have been anecdotal accounts and case studies that highlight the physiological changes that accompany a shift in personalities in people with DID. One of the most striking instances involves changes in the physical presentation of allergic reactions, visual acuity, and, relevantly, skin conditions.

The Case of the Disappearing Skin Problem
One particularly noteworthy case involved an individual who displayed different allergic responses and skin conditions based on which personality was dominant. When one personality was in control, the person exhibited severe skin problems. However, when another personality took over, the skin would clear up, and the issues would virtually disappear.

Scientific Insights
Such manifestations baffle medical understanding to some extent. The American Journal of Clinical Hypnosis has documented cases where one personality may be allergic to

a substance while another is not. Dr. Bennett Braun, who has reported on numerous DID cases, observed significant physiological changes between personalities, including changes in vision, handedness, voice, and the presence or absence of scars or skin conditions.

Possible Explanations

Psychosomatic Responses: The mind can influence the manifestation of physical symptoms. It's conceivable that, in certain DID cases, the psychological change between personalities causes a psychosomatic shift that can affect skin health.

Stress and Hormonal Changes: Different personalities might experience varying levels of stress or emotional states. Given that stress can exacerbate many skin conditions, a personality that is more relaxed or less prone to stress might exhibit clearer skin.

Neurological Mechanisms: The brain's chemistry and functioning can influence skin health. Changes in neural activity or neurotransmitter levels between personalities might play a role in the manifestation or absence of skin issues.

Personally, I have known people who have had certain conditions such as hay fever treated with hypnosis! It sounds crazy because one would think what has the mind got to do with hay fever which is a pollen problem?

Some alternative medicine practitioners believe that Psoriasis is a disease of sensitive people; of those who hide behind their skin and thus their own body makes a thicker skin.

For example, do sarcastic people, who are generally more sensitive, suffer more from Psoriasis?

Whilst this is a stretch for some of you who may suffer from Psoriasis, I personally believe there is some truth in this mind connection, particularly for some people.

For example, I believe that there is a Type A, that is more susceptible to having heart issues. This is the aggressive, domineering and impatient type.

There is also the type C, the nice person, that is more susceptible to Cancer.

Therefore there may well be a Type S, the sensitive type, who is more prone to skin issues.

Throughout history, physical symptoms and emotional states have often been intertwined. The face turning red with anger or going pale with fear are classic examples. One intriguing area of research explores the correlation between personality types, particularly those of sensitive individuals, and skin problems.

The Sensitive Soul: A Brief Overview
Highly sensitive people (HSP) are often more reactive to stimuli, both external and internal. They might be more affected by sensory details like loud noises or strong smells, as well as emotional events, making them more susceptible to stress responses.

Stress and the Skin: The Inextricable Link

Stress as a Trigger: Skin conditions like Psoriasis, eczema, and acne can be exacerbated by stress. Highly sensitive individuals often experience heightened stress reactions, potentially worsening or triggering these conditions.

Reference: Chida, Y., Mao, X. 2009. "Does psychosocial stress predict symptomatic herpes simplex virus recurrence? A meta-analytic investigation on prospective studies." Brain, Behavior, and Immunity.

Neurogenic Inflammation: The skin has its own immune and neuroendocrine system. When emotionally sensitive people face stressors, their response can trigger neurogenic inflammation in the skin.

Reference: Roosterman, D., Goerge, T., Schneider, S. W., Bunnett, N. W., & Steinhoff, M. 2006. "Neuronal control of skin function: The skin as a neuroimmunoendocrine organ." Physiological Reviews.

Psychodermatology: This field of dermatology focuses on the interaction between mind and skin. Emotional states, including those experienced more intensely by sensitive individuals, can influence skin conditions.

Reference: Gupta, M. A., & Gupta, A. K. 2003. "Psychodermatology: An update." Journal of the American Academy of Dermatology.


Other Personality Traits and Skin Connections

While sensitivity is a significant trait studied in relation to skin health, other personality aspects have been explored too:

Perfectionism: People who have perfectionistic tendencies may experience stress, anxiety, and depression, potentially affecting their skin health.

Reference: Ak, M., Lien, L., Sivertsen, B., Bjørngaard, J. H., & Ernstsen, L. 2021. "Perfectionism and incident acne: A population-based cohort study of young adults in Norway." PLoS ONE.

Anxiety and Depression: There's evidence that mood disorders can exacerbate skin conditions. The relationship is bi-directional: skin conditions can also lead to anxiety or depression, creating a vicious cycle.

Reference: Dalgard, F. J., Gieler, U., Tomas–Aragones, L., Lien, L., Poot, F., Jemec, G. B., ... & Szepietowski, J. C. 2015. "The psychological burden of skin diseases: a cross-sectional multicentre study among dermatological out-patients in 13 European countries." Journal of Investigative Dermatology.

How do you "undo" your personality for your Psoriasis to get better? You may be thinking, this is impossible!

Not exactly. Where there is a will, there is a way. Cognitive Behavioural Therapy (CBT), hypnotherapy and Neurolinguistic Programming (NLP) can help.

You can also try some Bach Flower Remedies from any decent health food shop in the modern world or by ordering online.

Please read up on these Bach Flower Remedies and see which one best suits you. You can take up to 5 at the same time:

Agrimony
Aspen
Centaury
Chicory
Holly
Walnut
Cremates
Crab Apple
Impatiens

You can put 1-2 drops of each under your tongue several times a day or mix 3-4 drops of each in a bottle of water and sip throughout the day.

Bach Flower Remedies have a gentle, yet very effective way of changing your weak personality traits.

## The link between intestinal health and neurological health

We have discussed how the mind can play a big role in affecting your skin. There is however a theory that goes the other way, where the gut and its health affect the mind!

There is a link between intestinal health and neurological health, suggesting that conditions often classified solely as mental or neurological could have their roots in gut health.

As mentioned in this book in various sections, a "Leaky gut", or increased intestinal permeability, refers to a condition where the walls of the intestine become less effective at filtering out unwanted particles. This allows substances, like toxins and bacteria, to pass into the bloodstream, potentially leading to systemic inflammation and immune reactions.

The gut-brain axis is a bidirectional communication system between the gastrointestinal tract and the nervous system. Recent research has highlighted how disruptions in gut health, including conditions like leaky gut, can influence brain function and behaviour.

It has been suggested that an imbalance in gut flora (dysbiosis) can lead to the production of harmful toxins. With a leaky gut, these toxins can enter the bloodstream and reach the brain, impacting its function.

Some alternative medicine practitioners suggest that conditions such as autism, ADHD, depression, and even schizophrenia could be influenced by gut health. They believe that by addressing gut dysbiosis and healing the intestinal lining, one can potentially alleviate some of the symptoms of these conditions.

The dietary approach is to restore a healthy balance of gut flora and repair the intestinal lining. This diet removes foods believed to contribute to gut dysbiosis and leaky gut, while introducing nutrient-rich foods that support healing.

Some practitioners also believe in the gut-brain connection in diseases like Epilepsy. The body is very much interconnected and ill health is not a one-sided thing. You need to address your "whole" body to get totally well; hence the term wholistic/holistic health.

Either way, it is important to be aware of the fact that your Psychology affects your gut and your Psoriasis and your gut health, affects your brain health.

References:
Cryan, J. F., & Dinan, T. G. (2012). Mind-altering microorganisms: the impact of the gut microbiota on brain and behaviour. Nature reviews neuroscience, 13(10), 701-712.

**Eczema**

I think it's important to mention Eczema in this book. Whilst similar in appearance, Eczema is thought by the medical profession to be a different problem to Psoriasis. Many alternative medicine practitioners do not share this view by the way!

People who have Eczema also usually have other related issues such as Asthma and they are interchangeable. Their asthma can get better but their Eczema gets worse and vice versa.

Eczema is a complicated disease, though personally I would say it is less complicated than Psoriasis, though I would say they are very similar. As with Psoriasis, a diary is extremely useful when it comes to treating Eczema. For example, I have seen many people totally get rid of their Eczema by eliminating something that was a red flag in their diary.

Examples of things that cause Eczema are: Eggs (huge culprit), chocolate and certain sweets, Ketchup, dairy products (especially milk and cheese) and wheat. For contact Eczema it can be things like Nickel or plastic.

Let's look a bit more in detail at Eczema and its differences to Psoriasis:

1. Eczema and Psoriasis definitions
Eczema (Atopic Dermatitis): Eczema is a chronic skin condition characterised by itchy, inflamed, and sometimes blistering skin. It often begins in childhood and can be triggered or worsened by various factors, including allergens, environmental conditions, and stress.

Psoriasis: As mentioned earlier, Psoriasis is an autoimmune disease wherein the body's immune system attacks healthy skin cells. This leads to the rapid buildup of skin cells on the surface, resulting in thick, scaly patches.

2. Appearance and Location
Eczema: Typically appears as dry, red, and itchy patches. These patches can become crusty, especially in areas like the insides of the elbows, back of the knees, and the neck.

Infected eczema may ooze and form crusts.

Psoriasis: Presents as red patches covered with thick, silvery scales. Commonly affects the knees, elbows, scalp, hands, feet, and lower back. In some cases, the nails may also be affected, leading to pitting or detachment.

3. Causes and Triggers

Eczema:

Causes: Exact causes are unclear but are believed to be a combination of genetic and environmental factors.

Triggers: Allergens (dust mites, pollen, mould), irritants (soaps, detergents), certain foods, stress, hormonal changes, and weather conditions.

Psoriasis:

Causes: Immune system dysfunction leading to inflammation and increased skin cell production.

Triggers: Infections, stress, certain medications, skin injuries (cuts, scrapes, bug bites), smoking, and excessive alcohol consumption and all the other things we have discussed thus far.

Reference: Boehncke, W. H., & Schön, M. P. 2015. "Psoriasis." Lancet.

4. Diagnosis

Eczema: Primarily diagnosed based on the appearance of the skin and patient history. Patch testing might be done to identify potential allergens.

Psoriasis: Diagnosis is often clinical, but a skin biopsy might be recommended to differentiate from other conditions.

5. Traditional Treatment

Eczema:

Topical treatments: Steroid creams, emollients, and calcineurin inhibitors.

Systemic treatments: Oral steroids, antihistamines, and immunosuppressants.

Phototherapy: Exposure to controlled amounts of natural or artificial light.

Psoriasis:

Topical treatments: Steroid creams, vitamin D analogs, coal tar, and tazarotene.

Systemic treatments: Methotrexate, cyclosporine, and biologics.

Phototherapy: Narrowband UVB light.

Reference: Lebwohl, M., et al. 2014. "US perspectives in the management of Psoriasis and Psoriatic arthritis: patient and physician results from the population-based Multinational Assessment of Psoriasis and Psoriatic Arthritis (MAPP) survey." American Journal of Clinical Dermatology.

6. Complications

Eczema: Chronic itching can lead to skin infections, scars, and sleep disturbances. The best remedy for itching is NOT to scratch it, as scratching brings more blood up to the skin. Use ice whenever you can; this is the best remedy for itching.

Psoriasis: Can be associated with Psoriatic arthritis, which affects the joints. It can also increase the risk of cardiovascular diseases, depression, and other conditions.

The reason why I mention Eczema here is that some people have both Eczema and Psoriasis and if not diagnosed properly, it can complicate things! At the end of the day, they are both issues with the internal system but Psoriasis is classified more as an auto-immune disorder by the medical community. Unlike Psoriasis, Eczema can also be caused by something external such as a metal bracelet or using the wrong shower gel (or any shower gel!).

Someone may have Psoriasis on their body but below their fingernails it may be Eczema and they may find that for example by removing eggs from their diet, the Eczema disappears but not their Psoriasis - or vice versa.

It is important to be sure what part of your skin lesions is which one out of Eczema or Psoriasis and a doctor can tell you this.

**Reflexology**

As a Reflexologist with over 30 years' experience, I cannot complete this book without reference to Reflexology.

Reflexology is an ancient practice rooted in the belief that different points on the feet, hands, and ears correspond to various organs and systems in the body. By applying pressure to these specific points, Reflexology aims to promote healing, alleviate tension, and restore balance in the body.

As discussed, Psoriasis is an autoimmune skin condition and will benefit from Reflexology through stimulation of certain key points, particularly the intestinal and liver points.

Reflexology is a complementary therapy grounded in the concept that the body is divided into ten longitudinal zones, each represented on the feet and hands. By manipulating specific zones, Reflexologists aim to stimulate energy pathways, enhance circulation, and support the body's natural healing processes.

Psoriasis is not just a superficial skin condition. As we have seen, research has shown links between gut health, liver function, and the severity of Psoriasis.

A growing body of evidence has shown that gut health, particularly the gut microbiome, may play a role in Psoriasis. Inflammation in the gut can lead to increased systemic inflammation, potentially exacerbating Psoriasis.

Reference: Salem, I., et al. 2018. "The Gut Microbiome as a Major Regulator of the Gut-Skin Axis." Frontiers in Microbiology.

The liver is crucial for detoxification. The liver is the orchestrator and detoxifier of your body. It is the liver that detoxifies chemicals and things like mould. Impaired liver function might lead to an accumulation of toxins, which could exacerbate skin conditions like Psoriasis.

Reference: Gisondi, P., et al. 2009. "Prevalence of liver disease in a cohort of Psoriatic patients treated with methotrexate and cyclosporine. A cross-sectional study." Dermatology.

Intestinal Points are located on the inner arch of the foot; basically the bottom half of both feet, the meaty part, the heel. Manipulating this area targets both the small and large intestines, which can promote better gut health and alleviate inflammation.

Liver Point is found on the right foot, located between the base of the fifth toe and the diaphragm line (midway up the foot). Stimulating this area aims to support liver function and detoxification.

While rigorous scientific research on Reflexology and Psoriasis is limited, proponents argue the following benefits:

Reduced Inflammation: By targeting the intestinal points, reflexology might help maintain a healthy gut lining, potentially reducing gut-related inflammation and its effects on Psoriasis.

Detoxification Support: Stimulating the liver point may aid in toxin removal, indirectly benefiting the skin.

Stress Reduction: Stress is a known trigger for Psoriasis flare-ups. Reflexology, in general, is lauded for its relaxation and stress-relieving properties.
Reference: Hernandez-Reif, M., et al. 2009. "Eczema Symptoms Reduced by Massage Therapy." Journal of Alternative and Complementary Medicine.

Is Reflexology the cure for Psoriasis? No it is not but it can definitely help flush your system out and re-balance you.

I have seen time and again that people with Psoriasis have tenderness and toxins sitting on the intestinal and liver Reflex points of the feet. In fact, I have never come across a Psoriasis sufferer that had clear feet Reflex points corresponding to the gut and liver.

In other words, when you press the liver and/or gut Reflex points located on the feet, the Psoriasis sufferer will jump up from pain. That says a lot! It is a clear sign that these points should at the very least be massaged once or twice daily. Ideally they should be worked on by a Reflexologist once a week in an intense manner.

For how to do Reflexology yourself, please refer to my other books such as The 10 Minute Back Pain Cure.

## Traditional medicine

Topical Corticosteroids: Widely prescribed, these potent anti-inflammatory drugs suppress the immune system, reducing inflammation and relieving associated itching. They're available in various strengths and formulations.

Vitamin D Analogues: These synthetic compounds are similar to vitamin D and help slow down the growth of skin cells. Examples include Calcipotriene and Calcitriol.

It is important to note here that these Vitamin D Analogues can seriously mark your skin (as mentioned already). They may get rid of your Psoriasis but you may end up with a much darker area on your skin where you have been applying the cream. This darker area is unlikely to disappear and can be aesthetically as distressing as Psoriasis lesions!
This is something that doctors don't tell you when they give you Vitamin D creams and whilst you will be grateful for their effects, you may end up regretting using them, especially if you overcome your Psoriasis yourself through the methods in this book.

Topical Retinoids: These are vitamin A derivatives like tazarotene that help reduce skin inflammation. They are often used in conjunction with other treatments.

Coal Tar: An older treatment method, coal tar reduces scaling, itching, and inflammation. It's available in various forms, including shampoos, creams, and oils.

Salicylic Acid: Available in both prescription and over-the-counter formulations, it helps promote the sloughing off of dead skin cells, reducing scaling.

Light Therapy (Phototherapy)
UVB Phototherapy: Exposes the skin to ultraviolet light B (UVB) to help slow the growth of affected skin cells.

Goeckerman Therapy: Combines UVB treatment with coal tar treatment.
Psoralen plus ultraviolet A (PUVA): After taking a light-sensitising drug, the skin is exposed to UVA light. It's effective but increases the risk for skin cancers! Seriously, it is sad to have such bad Psoriasis to have to go this route.

Laser Therapy: Excimer laser and pulsed dye laser treatments can target specific areas affected by mild to moderate Psoriasis.

Oral and Injected Medications
Methotrexate: An oral medication that suppresses the immune system and is also used for cancer and rheumatoid arthritis.

Cyclosporine: Immunosuppressant drug that inhibits the immune system's activity. It's similar to methotrexate but can affect kidney function and blood pressure. I would personally never do this no matter how bad my skin is!

Oral Retinoids: Acitretin is an oral retinoid that may be prescribed for severe cases of Psoriasis.

Biologics: Injected or infused drugs that target specific areas of the immune system. Examples include etanercept, infliximab, and adalimumab.

Apremilast (Otezla): An oral drug that works by suppressing an enzyme involved in inflammation.

As mentioned in the introduction of this book, you should not suddenly stop any medication whilst trying out the methods of this book.

This is especially so when it comes to oral steroids. They are very complicated and they do mess around with a great deal of your own body's systems. Suddenly coming off of them, even if your Psoriasis is getting better is not a good idea unless you are under medical supervision.

You can see that some of the above are very hardcore and come with a ton of their own side effects for sure. Some doctors recommend them so casually!

What you do with your body is your own choice at the end of the day. It is YOUR body! No doctor should have the right to tell you what to do with your own body or force you to do something that may cause other bigger problems such as cancer.

## Other things that help Psoriasis

We have covered a lot here already. As mentioned at the introduction, I have tried to stick to what really works and what has been scientifically shown to be at least relevant to Psoriasis.

However, if you want further assistance and are willing to try other "helpers", below is a list of them in no particular order.

Because Psoriasis is such a complicated disease, some of these will work better for some people than for others.

**Zinc - 50mg every day** - This is a very powerful mineral and very effective at combating Psoriasis. They say when you get stressed, the first mineral that disappears from your body is Zinc, so if you are particularly stressed, then a Zinc supplement may help you greatly. This is why I say some of these will work better for some people than others. Some people are more stressed than others!

Studies have shown that individuals with Psoriasis often have lower serum Zinc levels compared to healthy controls [3]. While it's unclear whether Zinc deficiency contributes to the onset of Psoriasis, it suggests that replenishing Zinc might be beneficial for those with the condition.
Reference: Burrows, N. P., Turnbull, A. J., Punchard, N. A., Thompson, R. P., & Jones, R. R. (1990). A trial of oral Zinc supplementation in Psoriasis. Cutis; cutaneous medicine for the practitioner, 46(1), 77-80.

Several studies have explored the use of topical Zinc treatments for Psoriasis. Zinc Pyrithione, for example, is an FDA-approved treatment for dandruff and has been shown to be effective in treating Psoriatic plaques. Its antifungal, anti-inflammatory, and antiproliferative properties might explain its efficacy [4]. This is why I recommend a shampoo with 2% Zinc Pyrithione.

Reference: Gupta, A. K., & Nicol, K. (2004). The use of sulfur in dermatology. Journal of Drugs in Dermatology: JDD, 3(4), 427-431.

There have been investigations into the effects of oral Zinc supplementation for Psoriasis management. My own experience has shown it is very beneficial for Psoriasis at around 50mg a day, at least for brief periods.

References:

[5] Michaëlsson, G., Ljunghall, K., & Danielson, B. G. (1993). Zinc in epidermis and dermis in healthy subjects. Acta Dermato-Venereologica, 73(4), 250-253.

[6] Burrows, N. P., Turnbull, A. J., Punchard, N. A., Thompson, R. P., & Jones, R. R. (1990). A trial of oral Zinc supplementation in Psoriasis. Cutis; cutaneous medicine for the practitioner, 46(1), 77-80.

As with any vitamin or mineral, make sure you buy a reputable brand.

By the way, many herbs and vitamins can make your Psoriasis worse! So don't go buying random things because you think they are good for you. Things like Echinacea, whilst good for the early stages of a cold, can make your Psoriasis worse.

**Omega 3 Fish Oil - 4000 mg a day** - Lots of people rave about the benefits of Omega 3s for Psoriasis and I have observed many positive benefits from supplementing with these.

Omega-3 and omega-6 are two primary types of polyunsaturated fatty acids. While both are essential for the body, the Western diet tends to be heavy on omega-6, which promotes inflammation, and light on omega-3, which has anti-inflammatory properties.

Eicosapentaenoic Acid (EPA) and Docosahexaenoic Acid (DHA) are the primary omega-3 fatty acids found in fish oil. These are the compounds that have been significantly linked to various health benefits, including improved skin health.

Reference: Simopoulos, A. P. 2002. "Omega-3 fatty acids in inflammation and autoimmune diseases." Journal of the American College of Nutrition.

Omega-3 fatty acids in fish oil can reduce the production of inflammatory cytokines and eicosanoids, potentially benefitting Psoriasis patients.

Reference: Calder, P. C. 2013. "Omega-3 polyunsaturated fatty acids and inflammatory processes: nutrition or pharmacology?" British Journal of Clinical Pharmacology.

Omega-3s can also support the skin's barrier function, helping retain moisture and keeping irritants out.

Immune Modulation: Given that Psoriasis is an autoimmune disorder, the immune-modulating effects of omega-3 fatty acids can be particularly relevant.

Reference: Ziboh, V. A., & Fletcher, M. P. 1992. "Dose-response effects of dietary gamma-linolenic acid-enriched oils on human polymorphonuclear-neutrophil biosynthesis of leukotriene B4." The American Journal of Clinical Nutrition.

Recommended Fish Oils for Psoriasis
Cold-Water Fish: Oils derived from cold-water fish, such as salmon, mackerel, herring, and sardines, are especially high in omega-3s and recommended for Psoriasis.

High EPA and DHA Content: Look for fish oils that have a high content of both EPA and DHA, as these are the most effective omega-3s. Make sure the fish oil is purified to eliminate potential contaminants.

Algal Oil: For vegetarians or those who avoid fish, algal oil (derived from algae) is a valuable source of DHA.
Reference: Swanson, D., Block, R., & Mousa, S. A. 2012. "Omega-3 fatty acids EPA and DHA: health benefits throughout life." Advances in Nutrition.

Dosage Recommendations
The exact amount of fish oil one should take for Psoriasis can vary based on individual needs, the severity of the condition, and the specific supplement's EPA and DHA content. However, some general guidelines exist:

General Health: For overall health, a dose of 250-500 mg combined EPA and DHA daily is often recommended.

Psoriasis and Other Inflammatory Conditions: Higher doses, ranging from 2 to 5 grams of combined EPA and

DHA daily, might be more effective for conditions like Psoriasis.

Reference: Søyland, E., Funk, J., Rajka, G., Sandberg, M., Thune, P., Rustad, L., ... & Middelfart, K. 1994. "Dietary supplementation with very long-chain n-3 fatty acids in patients with Psoriasis." New England Journal of Medicine.


**Curcumin or Turmeric Supplement** - Turmeric, a golden-hued spice native to Southeast Asia, has been a staple in traditional medicine systems for centuries. The active compound in turmeric, curcumin, has garnered significant attention for its anti-inflammatory, antioxidant, and therapeutic properties. Interestingly, cultures that regularly consume turmeric and curcumin in their diets often report fewer skin issues.

Before we delve into cultural observations, it's essential to understand turmeric and curcumin's basics:

Turmeric (Curcuma longa): A rhizomatous herbaceous perennial plant, turmeric is a member of the ginger family. Its roots are processed into the familiar yellow spice.

Curcumin: The primary active compound in turmeric, it's responsible for most of the spice's health benefits, particularly its anti-inflammatory and antioxidant effects.

Reference: Aggarwal, B. B., & Harikumar, K. B. 2009. "Potential therapeutic effects of curcumin, the anti-inflammatory agent, against neurodegenerative, cardiovascular, pulmonary, metabolic, autoimmune and neoplastic diseases." The International Journal of Biochemistry & Cell Biology.

Turmeric is an integral part of South Asian cuisine. It's used in curries, lentil soups, rice dishes, and even sweets. Anecdotal evidence and observational studies have shown that the prevalence of certain skin conditions might be lower in populations that consume turmeric regularly. Additionally, turmeric pastes have been traditionally used for skin treatments in Ayurveda, India's ancient medicinal system.

Reference: Thangapazham, R. L., Sharad, S., & Maheshwari, R. K. 2013. "Skin regenerative potentials of curcumin." Biofactors.

In countries like Thailand and Indonesia, turmeric is frequently used in traditional dishes and as a medicinal remedy. Similar to South Asia, these cultures exhibit fewer skin issues, potentially because of the protective effects of dietary turmeric.

With the rise in popularity of turmeric as a superfood in the West, there has been an increased interest in its potential benefits for skin health. While the consumption is not as deeply rooted culturally as in Asia, preliminary studies and anecdotal evidence suggest a positive impact on skin health for those who incorporate it into their diets.

Reference: Vaughn, A. R., Branum, A., & Sivamani, R. K. 2016. "Effects of turmeric (Curcuma longa) on skin health: A systematic review of the clinical evidence." Phytotherapy Research.

Curcumin has been shown to modulate several inflammatory pathways, helping to reduce skin conditions such as Psoriasis, Eczema, and Acne.

Reference: Menon, V. P., & Sudheer, A. R. 2007. "Antioxidant and anti-inflammatory properties of curcumin." Advances in Experimental Medicine and Biology.

Curcumin's ability to combat oxidative stress is well-documented. This property can protect the skin from damage, premature ageing, and other conditions exacerbated by free radicals.

Curcumin has been shown to accelerate the wound-healing process, reducing inflammation and oxidation, thus improving tissue repair.
Reference: Tejada, S., Manayi, A., Daglia, M., Nabavi, S. F., Sureda, A., Hajheydari, Z., ... & Nabavi, S. M. 2016. "Wound healing effects of curcumin: A short review." Current Pharmaceutical Biotechnology.

Cultures that have embraced turmeric and curcumin in their diets for generations might be reaping more than just culinary rewards. Their skin health, potentially enhanced by the regular consumption of this golden spice, serves as an intriguing testament to the potential benefits of dietary choices on overall health. As modern science catches up with ancient wisdom, the incorporation of turmeric into diets worldwide may become more than just a trend - it might become a universally recommended staple for skin vitality.

You can either start adding Curcumin or Turmeric to your food or take a good high quality supplement. Take the recommended amount and see how you get on. You may want to increase or decrease it according to results.

One of my friends has a lot of issues with his joints and chronic arthritis and he religiously takes several grams of Turmeric daily. When he takes the Turmeric, he has no joint issues!

I have witnessed many Psoriasis sufferers get better with relatively high doses of Turmeric but it does not work for everyone and can give tummy issues. Start slow and see how it goes.


**Prebiotics and probiotics** - Unless you have been living under a rock, you would have heard these two fad names. But are they fads? More and more scientists are jumping on the pre and probiotic bandwagon and putting down a whole load of diseases to lack of prebiotic or probiotics or both.

Gut health has taken centre stage in many health discussions over recent years, leading to an increased interest in prebiotics and probiotics. A mounting body of evidence suggests that the health of our gut can have a profound influence on our skin. This article will explore the world of prebiotics and probiotics, their presence in food, and their potential link to skin conditions like Psoriasis.

Prebiotics: These are non-digestible fibres and compounds that promote the growth of beneficial gut bacteria. Essentially, they act as food for probiotics.
Reference: Gibson, G. R., Hutkins, R., Sanders, M. E., Prescott, S. L., Reimer, R. A., Salminen, S. J., ... & Reid, G. 2017. "The International Scientific Association for Probiotics

and Prebiotics (ISAPP) consensus statement on the definition and scope of prebiotics." Nature Reviews Gastroenterology & Hepatology.

Probiotics: These are live beneficial bacteria that, when consumed in adequate amounts, can provide health benefits, particularly for the digestive system.
Reference: Hill, C., Guarner, F., Reid, G., Gibson, G. R., Merenstein, D. J., Pot, B., ... & Calder, P. C. 2014. "The International Scientific Association for Probiotics and Prebiotics consensus statement on the scope and appropriate use of the term probiotic." Nature Reviews Gastroenterology & Hepatology.

Food Sources

Prebiotics:
Vegetables: Garlic, onions, leeks, asparagus, and Jerusalem artichokes.
Grains: Barley, oats, and wheat.
Fruits: Apples, bananas, and berries.
Others: Flaxseeds and seaweed.

Probiotics:
Fermented Dairy: Yogurt and kefir.
Fermented Vegetables: Sauerkraut, kimchi, and pickles.
Fermented Soy: Miso and tempeh.
Beverages: Kombucha and certain fermented drinks.

A growing body of evidence highlights a link between gut health and skin conditions. Let's look at how imbalances in the gut microbiome could affect skin health.

An imbalanced gut can lead to increased systemic inflammation, potentially exacerbating inflammatory skin conditions like Psoriasis.

Reference: Salem, I., Ramser, A., Isham, N., & Ghannoum, M. A. 2018. "The gut microbiome as a major regulator of the gut-skin axis." Frontiers in Microbiology.

A compromised gut lining can increase permeability, allowing harmful substances to enter the bloodstream, which might influence skin health.

Reference: Odenwald, M. A., & Turner, J. R. 2017. "The intestinal epithelial barrier: a therapeutic target?" Nature Reviews Gastroenterology & Hepatology.

Gut imbalances can modulate immune responses, potentially triggering or exacerbating autoimmune skin conditions like Psoriasis.

Reference: Tan, L., Zhao, S., Zhu, W., Wu, L., Li, J., Shen, M., ... & Chen, X. 2018. "The Akkermansia muciniphila is a gut microbiota signature in Psoriasis." Experimental Dermatology.

The significance of prebiotics and probiotics in maintaining gut equilibrium cannot be understated. Through their role in fostering a balanced gut microbiome, they may influence skin health and conditions like Psoriasis. As research in this area continues to burgeon, understanding the gut-skin connection may pave the way for novel therapeutic interventions.

There is no doubt that in certain circumstances, a lack of prebiotics or probiotics can cause Psoriasis to kick off or cause it to not calm down. For example, if you have just had a heavy dose of antibiotics, you may have developed Psoriasis for the first time. Or your Psoriasis may have gotten worse as a result of taking antibiotics.

The discovery of antibiotics revolutionised medicine, saving countless lives and effectively combating bacterial infections. However, as with most powerful tools, antibiotics come with caveats. One of the most notable is their effect on our gut flora, the community of microorganisms that reside in our intestines. This article delves into the impact of antibiotics on this critical microbiome, the importance of judicious antibiotic use, and methods to restore gut health post-treatment.

While antibiotics are designed to kill harmful bacteria causing infections, they can't always differentiate between pathogenic bacteria and the beneficial bacteria that inhabit our gut.

Disruption of Gut Balance: Antibiotics can deplete both harmful and beneficial bacteria. This can lead to a disrupted microbial balance, termed dysbiosis.

Reference: Jernberg, C., Löfmark, S., Edlund, C., & Jansson, J. K. 2007. "Long-term ecological impacts of antibiotic administration on the human intestinal microbiota." The ISME Journal.

Dysbiosis can manifest in various ways, from transient diarrhea to conditions like Clostridioides difficile infection, which can be severe and life-threatening.

Post-antibiotic recovery is essential for restoring the gut's microbiome. As I mentioned earlier, my own Psoriasis was kicked off with several courses of antibiotics given to me for something or another!

There  are ways to aid the process of replenishing gut flora.

Probiotics: Consuming live beneficial bacteria can help restore the gut flora. Probiotics can be found in fermented foods like yogurt, kefir, sauerkraut, kimchi, and kombucha or in supplement form.
Reference: Hickson, M. 2011. "Probiotics in the prevention of antibiotic-associated diarrhoea and Clostridium difficile infection." Therapeutic Advances in Gastroenterology.

Prebiotics: These non-digestible fibres and compounds feed the beneficial bacteria, promoting their growth and activity. Foods rich in prebiotics include garlic, onions, leeks, asparagus, and bananas.

Diverse Diet: A varied diet rich in whole foods, fruits, and vegetables can foster a diverse microbiome, which is resilient and beneficial for health.
Reference: David, L. A., Maurice, C. F., Carmody, R. N., Gootenberg, D. B., Button, J. E., Wolfe, B. E., ... & Turnbaugh, P. J. 2014. "Diet rapidly and reproducibly alters the human gut microbiome." Nature.
Judicious Use of Antibiotics

It's essential to appreciate the power and potential pitfalls of antibiotics:

Antibiotics can't treat viral infections. They're often inappropriately prescribed for conditions like colds and the flu, where they offer no benefit.

***Antibiotics do nothing for <u>viral</u> conditions!***

Reference: Fleming-Dutra, K. E., Hersh, A. L., Shapiro, D. J., Bartoces, M., Enns, E. A., File Jr, T. M., ... & Hicks, L. A. 2016. "Prevalence of inappropriate antibiotic prescriptions among US ambulatory care visits, 2010-2011." JAMA.

When prescribed, it's crucial to take the entire course as directed, even if you feel better, to ensure all pathogenic bacteria are eradicated and to reduce the risk of antibiotic resistance.

While sometimes essential, frequent antibiotic use can lead to antibiotic resistance and harm the gut flora.
Reference: Costelloe, C., Metcalfe, C., Lovering, A., Mant, D., & Hay, A. D. 2010. "Effect of antibiotic prescribing in primary care on antimicrobial resistance in individual patients: systematic review and meta-analysis." BMJ.

### Healing crisis

You may have heard this term before. If Vitamin D supplementation and a water softener have not sufficiently alleviated your Psoriasis and you are having to go the extra route of changing your diet to a more vegetarian one, eliminating certain foods such as saturated fats, junk, sugars etc and trying Intermittent Fasting, then you may experience an initial Healing Crisis.

Healing Crisis is when the body goes into detox mode and you may get things happening which don't usually occur with your body. Depending on the individual, it can be anything: headaches, worsting of skin issues (including Psoriasis!), excess gas, bloating, bad breath, tiredness, joint aches, pains and many other things.

This is normal and a sign that your body is detoxifying. If it is too much to take, you may want to ease up on whatever you are doing but don't let this temporary healing crisis put you off. It is a sign that things are going in the right way.

A healing crisis, often referred to as the Herxheimer reaction, is a temporary exacerbation of symptoms during the detoxification or healing process. This reaction is believed to occur when the body releases stored toxins, leading to a temporary spike in symptoms.

Characteristics of a Healing Crisis:
Intensified Symptoms: One might experience a sudden and temporary increase in the severity of their psoriasis or other symptoms.

Additional Symptoms: These can range from flu-like symptoms, fatigue, headache, joint pains, night sweats, and other detox reactions.

Emotional Release: Some individuals report mood swings or feelings of anxiety or depression during a healing crisis.

Duration and Variability
The duration of a healing crisis varies widely among individuals. It can last anywhere from a day to, more rarely, a few weeks. The length and intensity often depend on several factors:

Individual Toxin Load: Those with a higher load of toxins might experience a more intense or prolonged healing crisis.

Detox Method: More aggressive detox methods can lead to a more pronounced healing crisis.

Overall Health: Individual health status and resilience can influence the body's response and recovery time.

Is a Healing Crisis a Good Sign?
The healing crisis is often interpreted as a sign that the body is effectively eliminating toxins and beginning to heal. Proponents argue that once the healing crisis subsides, individuals experience a marked improvement in their condition and overall well-being.

However, it's essential to approach this phenomenon with caution. Not all worsening symptoms indicate a healing crisis; they could be signs of a negative reaction or other health issues. It's crucial to consult with a healthcare provider when considering detox strategies or if experiencing worsening symptoms.

Generally, a Healing Crisis, as hard as it is, lasts for a few short days.

Something else to look for if you are going to do a more detox diet is your tongue. Have a look at your tongue in the mirror at the outset. You may find different coloured areas or your tongue looking patchy and not smooth. What you will find after a few months of changing your diet and eliminating the offending foods, is a more smooth and even tongue, which is a big clue as to your general health.

If you have taken a variety of different foods such as dairy and wheat out of your diet, you may want to take a good multivitamin-mineral tablet to ensure you are not deficient of some essential ones.

Once your healing crisis is over and you begin healing, you may well notice healing of many other ailments. For example I have seen people who have given top wheat see a total elimination of their Blepharitis, IBS, dermatitis etc

As a general rule, it takes about 2 months to see substantial changes and to start getting better, especially if you have stubborn Psoriasis. Even a slice of bread can take up to 2 months to fully clear the body.

## Conclusion

Well done! You have made it to the end of the book. That is an achievement in itself.

You are the one that will decide to what extent, if any you want your Psoriasis gone and how much of this book you will put into practice.

Whilst we all claim to want perfect health, we are often not willing to pay the price for it, in terms of inconveniences and changes in habit and lifestyle. In addition, most health issues are stubborn and "fight back"! You need to be persistent and remember that you will have bad days but as long as you keep going in the right direction, you will get there.

I understand that many of you will be skeptical too and may not want to put the principles of this book into practice. However, try them before knocking them.

Some people learn to live with their diseases or are not as bothered as some others. A minority even feel lost without their signature disease! I am serious!

At the highest level will be someone that really wants their Psoriasis gone and they will put all the principles in this book immediately into practice AND continue to stick to them for life. They are highly likely to become and remain Psoriasis-free for life.

Another person may try all or some of the principles for a while or periodically, to be partially or wholly Psoriasis-free for a while.

There will also be the person reading some or all of this book and practicing one or none of the suggestions for their own reasons.

If there is one thing I have learnt as a complimentary medicine practitioner, employer and entrepreneur is that every person is different and one cannot predict how a person will behave. I cannot also force you to behave in a certain manner for the long term.

Big decisions always have to come from the person and with a valid reason behind them. If the reason is not valid enough, the chances are that the person will not stick to that decision long term.

For example, the single (unmarried) Psoriasis sufferer may have a lot more reason and motivation for practising what is laid out in this book that the married person who feels they no longer need to look their best to attract a partner!

Whatever your choice, good luck with it. You will not be judged but please remember that as and when you are serious about ridding yourself of Psoriasis, please come back to this book.

For everyone else who is happy to have found this book and determined enough to put its principles into practice,

the best of luck to you and remember, persistence and a
positive mind always pay off.

All the best.


Parham Donyai